Belly Dance
for Health,
Happiness and
Empowerment

Belly Dance for Health, Happiness and Empowerment

Tina Hobin

AYNI
BOOKS

Winchester, UK
Washington, USA

First published by Ayni Books, 2015
Ayni Books is an imprint of John Hunt Publishing Ltd., Laurel House, Station Approach,
Alresford, Hants, SO24 9JH, UK
office1@jhpbooks.net
www.johnhuntpublishing.com
www.ayni-books.com

For distributor details and how to order please visit the 'Ordering' section on our website.

Text copyright: Tina Hobin 2014

ISBN: 978 1 78279 917 7
Library of Congress Control Number: 2015930749

A CIP catalogue record for this book is available from the British Library.

Design: Stuart Davies

Printed and bound by CPI Group (UK) Ltd, Croydon, CR0 4YY, UK

We operate a distinctive and ethical publishing philosophy in all
areas of our business, from our global network of authors to
production and worldwide distribution.

CONTENTS

There was a star danced
And under that was I born.
(*Much Ado About Nothing*, 1598–9, Act 2 Scene 1)

Why would you or anyone else wish to take up belly dancing?
Why does it attract people from all walks of life?
How can a sportsman benefit as much from this original and
sensual dance as a pregnant woman?
And how can you wiggle your way to a beautiful body, mind
and soul?
Why not wrap yourself up in the enticing world of oriental
dance, which has tremendous emotional appeal and grace. Let
the music envelop your mind, body and soul, and feel the
unique movements of this ancient art-form work wonders
around your midriff.
(Nikki Hobin)

Introduction

The Healing Power of the Belly Dance

The belly dance evolved from magic and secular dances, fertility and childbirth rituals, mourning and festivities. From its earliest beginnings centuries ago to the present day, women from all cultures have embraced this quintessential sacred dance. Like no other dance this ancient art, specifically related to women, can stimulate the unconscious, embody natural healing powers, aid spiritual growth and restore harmony and balance. The rotating, rolling and thrusting movements of the abdominal and pelvic region which have been passed down from generation to generation over the centuries are especially significant, as the abdomen which is accentuated in the dance is an extremely important part of the body, the seat of all sexual and child-bearing activities. The purpose of these specific movements in ancient cultures was to encourage sexual stimulation, the original aim being to initiate coitus (sexual intercourse). The birth dance, which is believed to have originated in pre-biblical times, facilitated birthing and celebrated the birth and motherhood.

Over the years there has been a dramatic increase in the popularity of the belly dance in the UK and overseas, not only as a beautiful art form but as a unique form of exercise that has tremendous healing qualities both psychologically and physiologically.

In contrast to other conventional dance forms and exercise which impose movement upon the individual, this ancient dance forms an intrinsic power within one which imposes self-expression, creativity and femininity, boosts energy levels, and although it cannot be claimed that belly dancing is a cure for all, it does help to stimulate the body's healing process.

Unlike other forms of dance and exercise the movements of the belly dance are based on the natural structure of the body and are a natural, safe and effective way of achieving help to move the body as it is designed to move, without any stress or strain, and this is why it is so beneficial to everyone irrespective of age, size, health or fitness levels.

This low-impact, weight-bearing, gentle, unique form of exercise will enable you to make full use of your muscles in a proper and co-ordinated way which will help to improve muscle tone, in particular the core muscles and those that surround and support internal organs. The movements of the dance also focus on 'isolations' which enable you to move groups of muscles independently.

The moves also stretch and strengthen the pelvic floor, massage internal organs, help to maintain a healthy cardiovascular system, lessen tension and depression, improve co-ordination, balance and flexibility, improve posture, and ease low back pain. Although it cannot be claimed that belly dancing is a cure for all ills, the movements of the dance can without a doubt help those with IBS and other digestive problems. Learners with the early stages of endometriosis also found they gained great relief from doing the movements that concentrated on the abdomini. It has also helped those with the early stages of arthritis, fibromyalgia and dementia. Recently there has been a lot of research done on the benefits of dance for those with dementia, and for others it has helped to improve the intimate side of their life, both for themselves and their partners.

Learning to belly dance has also helped those who suffer from other digestive problems, relieved menstrual and menopausal problems, and aided many other health and fitness issues.

As you read through the following pages you will become aware of the benefits of this very unique form of exercise. You will also understand the root causes of illnesses and how, by embracing this empowering dance once practised by ancient cultures, you can stimulate your body's natural healing power and achieve self-improvement, happiness, harmony, health, vitality and empowerment.

Part I

The Importance of Exercise

The Belly Dance – Dance of Life

The truest expression of a people is in its dances and its music.
Bodies never lie.
(*New York Times Magazine*, 11 May 1975)

Dance is the language of life, the oldest form of communication in the universe, the essence of which awakens the soul, stimulates the unconscious and embodies natural healing powers. The earthy quintessence of this sacred dance potentially embraces the awakening of feminine consciousness and reconciliation with the divine feminine principle, restoring harmony and balance within the universe.

This ancient art form perpetuates a new passage of spirituality and enlightenment, which channels both physical and creative energies. Its natural rhythm provides emotions of joy, happiness and satisfaction, and enables you to express yourself through freedom of movement.

Managing the Mind and Spiritual Well-Being – Spiritual Enlightenment

1. The healing journey

It is exercise alone that supports the spirits and keeps the mind in vigour.
(Cicero)

Irrespective of age, correct exercise in reasonable amounts is good physically and mentally for everyone. Just as babies and children need plenty of exercise to encourage sturdy development, adults also need to continue with appropriate exercise in order to maintain fitness levels, improve mobility and weight control, lessen fatigue, improve one's quality of sleep, and develop an overall sense of well-being. Lack of exercise is a common cause of being overweight, having poor posture, experiencing breathlessness, lethargy, premature ageing, weakness of muscles and stiff joints.

Gentle and sustained dance movement increases the capacity and interchange of oxygen in the lungs, which helps the whole body to function well. It promotes lower total cholesterol levels and higher levels of good cholesterol. It lessens and dispels hormone chemicals which accumulate in the body in times of stress.

Exercise is not only for the young, the fit and the healthy, but also for those of you who are reaching middle age, the elderly, or those whose ability to exercise is restricted owing to injury or medical problems. Many people who suffer from pain and discomfort are reluctant to exercise through ignorance or fear, which is understandable. But whatever the problem, it is vitally important to do some form of gentle exercise such as belly dancing, ballroom dancing, walking or other low-impact exercise. I should mention at this point that 'low impact' means to exercise without putting any stress on your bones or joints, for example not jarring your body on a hard surface as in jogging, jumping up and down, or over-stretching. Low-impact exercise is much more beneficial than strenuous and high-impact exercise for some conditions.

Middle-aged and elderly people are inclined to be physically inactive, and as a result become prone to the debilitating effects of inactivity that threaten an independent lifestyle. As we get older, joints get drier, become stiff, and lose their range of mobility, and as a result, restrict movement. Muscles lose their elasticity and strength, and become weak. The maintenance of muscle strength is extremely important for maintaining the functions of the body, for example, a healthy cardiovascular and respiratory system, posture, balance and co-ordination, all of which help retain basic physical skills.

As the years tick by, taking part in low-impact physical daily activities and practising correct breathing techniques will help to increase the blood flow and rise in oxygen levels to your brain; this will provide mental stimulation for your brain cells, which is crucial to your well-being and independence.

2. The healing process

Self-image

In quietness and in your confidence shall be your strength. (Isaiah 30:15)

Belly dancing is a non-discriminate dance form which can be enjoyed equally by both sexes, from the age of 3 to 83 plus. People with special needs and those suffering from mental or physical problems have also benefited from this therapeutic dance, as have the most active sportsmen, women and children. Size is of no importance. A larger woman is of equal fascination in her movements as a young girl with a perfect figure. Unfortunately women in the West are constantly subjected to some kind of media influence on self-image and a growing amount of pressure to look much slimmer and younger than their actual age. As a result they become so absorbed with their self-image they have excessive cosmetic surgery; some people even take drastic measures to look like their idol.

That sort of perfection is not only unnatural but costs a fortune to achieve. Today everything seems to be about exposing one's sexuality, which is very unhealthy and, as a result of media coverage that encourages this attitude, ordinary women become dissatisfied with themselves, believing they are too fat, or too thin, their bottoms are too big, boobs too small, they have frown lines or too many wrinkles. And because women feel unattractive, their acceptance of themselves becomes negative, and as a result physical and emotional dysfunction manifests itself in the form of depression, irritability, lethargy and low self-esteem.

It certainly doesn't help when celebrities and stars of stage and screen are constantly featured in newspapers and magazines with headlines like, "Don't they look fantastic for their age!" and describing them as beautiful, when in fact they have had numerous procedures done to achieve that perfect body and flawless face. Some celebrities promote fitness books and DVDs, but no matter how dedicated you become and follow their fitness regimes, you will never achieve their looks unless you have the same cosmetic procedures.

I recently asked sixty men and women what their perception of a beautiful female body was. Fifty-seven men said: a curvaceous, voluptuous, wholesome body (no surprise there), and three men thought Marilyn Monroe, Keira Knightley and Brigitte Bardot had perfect bodies. However, all the men agreed that breast implants, long artificial eyelashes and expressionless faces due to Botox and fillers were very unattractive and not at all sexy.

Not surprisingly the women had very different perceptions of a beautiful female body and said: being tall and slender, toned in all the right places, having grace, poise, character and warmth, inner strength, a wonderful personality, confidence and a lovely smile, a shapely body, being a natural woman and knowing how to wear the right clothes to flatter their figure.

There are numerous natural, sensuous and beautiful-looking women, including many famous ones who radiate a special aura because they accept their lines and wrinkles with pride and confidence as they age, and are still attractive, sensual, and have sex appeal.

Beauty and sensuality come from within and have little to do with how big your boobs are, the length of your eyelashes, or how perfect your face looks.

Mums who encourage their young daughters to wear make-up and designer clothes and strut around emulating their favourite celebrities, or encourage them to enter dance competitions, all made up and wearing exotic sequined costumes as they attempt to gyrate sexually like some pop star, are so deluded. Instead of encouraging their daughters and bringing them up to behave like normal 10-year-old youngsters, these misguided mums are making decisions that could lead to dire psychological problems for their child. Childhood is very precious and their innocence should be protected. How satisfied will they be with their looks, body and their sexuality in a few years' time?

Acceptance of ourselves the way we are is vitally important to our well-being. In belly dancing our emotions surface, giving us the opportunity to connect with ourselves and explore our basic instincts, for example, our sexual energy and feminine source. It also helps us to be realistic in our expectations of ourselves mentally, physically and spiritually.

Even learners who have been subjected to sexual abuse have been able to get in touch and accept their bodies through the belly dance, which has channelled their negative emotions in a more positive way.

In belly dancing you can aim to achieve self-confidence and self-esteem, be happy about the way you are, and value yourself as a human being. Once you have discovered yourself through the belly dance, you will achieve self-improvement, harmony and balance.

Throughout history this sacred dance has been a powerful means through which women expressed and celebrated their divine femininity, sexual energy and fertility. The belly dance also has the effect of enhancing your sex life in many subtle ways. You become aware of your newly acquired sensuality and sexuality, confidence, suppleness and vitality, through the body's natural movements, all of which combine to heighten love-making for yourself and your partner, so bringing about a new dimension of communication and pleasure to your relationship. A new woman reborn through the belly dance is a beautiful, vital, sensual and happy being.

Many years ago, a more senior learner who was attending one of my weekly workshops had been widowed for many, many years and since her husband's death had never embarked on another relationship. One morning she came to see me before we started the day, to tell me, with a huge grin on her face, about an experience she had had. What transpired was that she awoke during the night to find that her sexual responsiveness which had been suppressed for all those years, was suddenly re-awakened and released; in her own words she said everything was "going like the clappers for hours" and all she could do was pace the floor all night. Trying to keep my face straight was an effort as I explained that that was absolutely fantastic and had happened because, through the movements of the dance, she had got in touch with her sexuality again. She couldn't wait to tell some of the others in the group what she had experienced and they too thought it was hilarious, but great. Sometime later I heard that she was in a relationship with a lovely man and life was great again.

3. Spirituality through the belly dance

The means by which we live have outdistanced the ends for which we live. Our scientific power has outrun our spiritual power. We have guided missiles and misguided men.
(Martin Luther King, *Strength to Love*, 1963, ch. 7)

Getting in touch with one's inner spirituality through the creative energies of the belly dance has significant healing values on a spiritual, psychological and physical level. Energising both nerves and muscles (the neuromuscular system) through the dance produces physical and mental changes. This is a process of healing which stimulates the conscious and unconscious, decreases negative emotions, and improves self-perception – changes that will nurture and nourish your whole being, restore balance and harmony, creating a sense of inner peace, happiness and spiritual enlightenment.

In matriarchal societies, dance rituals were a spiritual channel through which the great earth goddess, the sacred feminine and symbol of life, death and rebirth, embraced and celebrated woman's femininity in its entirety.

Without spirituality we are incomplete. Inner spirituality stimulates the unconscious, cultivates our inner growth, creates harmony and unity with life's forces and communication with the divine, helping us to understand our inner feelings and life itself.

Sadly, in today's modern world people of all ages are living with little restraint, becoming more concerned with the material-istic values of life. Obsessed with the latest hi-tech gadgets, individuals are becoming more obsessed about their looks, owning more possessions than they can actually cope with or appreciate. Shallow, selfish, arrogant, ignorant and irresponsible people have little or no self-discipline, with respect neither for themselves, other people, or authority. It is also very worrying that very young children are becoming disrespectful, disruptive, undisciplined and violent due to lack of parental control and inept teachers.

Inner peace achieves emotional balance, increases tolerance, develops a sense of self-respect and a state of fulfilment. Recognise your weaknesses and your strengths. Listen to your mind and be aware of how your body feels; don't be afraid to get in touch with your feelings or be unwilling to change. It will not be easy, but try to be positive and find the correct way to deal with your problems.

Not only is love a great healer but it is also a powerful force. A true love within a marriage or partnership benefits each individual, both physically and mentally, and brings stability within the relationship and family. There are many different types of love – for self, and others.

Open up your heart and learn to love yourself, because if you don't love yourself, you cannot love others. Without love, there will never be a state of peaceful and harmonious co-existence among mankind. I believe the reason for our existence on this earth plane is to love, procreate and spread peace.

The very first religion was believed to be preconceived by women for women, and religious rituals in dance were a means of celebrating the sacred feminine force, the symbol of wholeness and source of all life on earth.

The expression of the divine feminine and veneration of women primarily diminished as Christianity, Islam and other religions gradually emerged. Dominance and suppression by male hierarchies totally denied women their sexual freedom, creativity and spiritual powers, and condemned them as being evil seductresses to all men. Sexually humiliated, bullied and under constant threat of punishment, women became subservient to men, and as a result feminine empowerment diminished. Sadly, in some parts of the world women still are subservient to men.

For centuries women have been cut off from this original source, but through this ancient dance we all have the potential to search our souls, find spiritual enlightenment and gain personal empowerment. Through these creative energies we can unite and renew life's forces and redeem the veneration of the divine feminine, return to our natural source, restore and balance universal harmony, and play a decisive role in reconciling humanity again with the great Earth Mother.

4. Stress

We think of strength, growth and spiritual healing
And a time for planting our energies.
(Ed McGaa Eagle Man, *Mother Earth Spirituality*)

Stress has become a major health problem which can have long-term effects on our bodies and mental stability, weakening our body's defences against diseases. Stress is the second biggest cause of illness in the workplace, and absenteeism costs industry billions of pounds a year, excluding the incalculable costs of loss of efficiency.

Stress can be caused by the inability to cope with the pressures experienced in modern-day living and in the workplace. Life-changing situations, such as the loss of a loved one, the break-up of a relationship, divorce or losing your job, being a perfectionist or controlling, an illness or just life in general can cause great stress.

Signs of stress can be tendencies towards tiredness, anxiety and tension, irritability, indecision and anger, being weepy, loss of concentration, and a loss of humour, a feeling of sickness in the stomach, severe headaches and for some people migraine. An increase in smoking and drinking alcohol can also be stress-related symptoms. It's very important to lessen your intake of alcohol and cut down on the number of cups of coffee you drink in a day and the cigarettes you smoke as they only contribute to raising your stress levels, not lowering your stress levels.

Stress is a powerful force and unless these symptoms are treated, more serious medical problems such as coronary heart disease, high blood pressure, peptic ulcers, digestive problems, depression or a nervous breakdown may develop.

Although stress cannot be completely avoided, the majority of us do manage to survive a certain amount of stress, which, according to specialists in this field, is good for us. However, it is difficult to define the literal meaning of stress, as it means something different to each and every one of us.

It is important to find ways of managing your stress. Take stock, and really think seriously about the probable causes and symptoms of your stress, and its influence on your behaviour, physically and mentally. It may help you to make a list of all the things that you think may be causing you stress, and if possible tackle the cause. Think carefully about your priorities. Look at your goals, short and long term, and recognise your abilities and limitations. Accept what you cannot change, then learn to adapt to what you cannot change. Be aware that your stress can also affect everyone around you at home and in the workplace.

The ability to relax is an important factor in helping to relieve stress; exercising and developing new interests are all essential elements in countering stress and relieving tension and depression. Belly dancing can be very beneficial in all these areas. This wonderful form of exercise, combined with correct breathing techniques, will release those natural chemicals called endorphins which will help reduce tension and depression, raise your energy levels and stamina, tone up your body and help you feel more confident and positive in self-image. When you learn the breathing techniques on page 61 and the art of relaxation on page 102, you will help to reduce your stress levels, and as a result your health and general well-being will benefit.

Remember, too much stress can have a negative effect on your health and general well-being, so it is very important to seek the right treatment for your needs if you cannot cope. If you feel that your stress is getting out of control, do seek advice from your doctor or a counsellor.

For advice on how to manage stress, contact info@stress.org.uk

Fighting Illness

5. Importance of dance for dementia and Alzheimer's

Researcher and neurologist Joe Verghese at the Albert Einstein College of Medicine, New York, conducted a study of eleven physical activities on people who were 75 years of age and found that dancing was the only one that was associated with a lower risk of dementia.

A 21-year-old study published in the *New England Journal of Medicine* has also found that dancing can lower the risk of Alzheimer's and other forms of dementia in elderly people.

Alexander Chancellor's article in *Saga*, October 2003, stated that researchers in the US found that dancing lowers the risk of older people developing Alzheimer's disease and other forms of dementia by a dramatic 76%.

I believe this is not only because of the physical effort dancing entails, but also because circulation is improved and levels of oxygen to the brain are increased which calms down a dementia patient's moods and creates a feeling of general well-being.

While in Australia, I came across an article in *The Australian Women's Weekly*, December 2009, about recent research from Tufts University in Boston, USA, which showed that exercising for about 30 minutes a day, three days a week, can induce neurogenesis, the formation of new neurons, cells which are a special type of cell in the body described as building blocks which help your learning and memory ability. Aged 55 or 95, it's never too late to put on the dancing shoes, whether it's belly or ballroom dancing. Over the years I have done several belly-dancing sessions with groups of people who have dementia and, combined with correct breathing techniques, it has been a very beneficial exercise as it helped to calm them down, keep them fit and have some fun while learning.

If you find that you are having problems with your memory,

you can help to boost your brain power by including fish oils in your diet. Omega 3 fatty acids found in oily fish such as sardines, tuna, salmon and mackerel are believed to be a vital source in helping the elderly to improve and maintain their memory.

The term 'dementia' is used to describe symptoms that occur when the brain is affected by certain diseases and conditions. Many problems occur which include: a lack of understanding, confusion, loss of memory and difficulties with speech and co-ordination, and mood changes.

If you have any concerns about Alzheimer's or dementia, contact the helpline for support and information on 0845 300 0336 in the UK; or from overseas +44 (0)207 423 3500. Or email enquiries@alzheimers.org.uk

6. Belly dancing and ill health

Look at your health; if you have it, praise God and value it next to a good conscience, for health is the second blessing that we mortals are capable of that money cannot buy.
(*The Compleat Angler*, 1653, Part I, ch. 21)

The most important thing in illness is never to lose heart.
(Nikolai Lenin)

Over the years, I have had women attending classes with the following illnesses: the early stages of multiple sclerosis, endometriosis, arthritis, osteoporosis, chronic fatigue syndrome, fibromyalgia, two learners with cystic fibrosis, IBS, colitis, asthma, digestive problems, obesity, tension, depression or bipolar disorder (a mental illness which used to be described as manic depression), heart and poor circulatory problems, and those who have had cancer or a hysterectomy. Even the deaf have attended classes and learnt to follow the rhythms by feeling the vibrations of the music through the floor. Partially blind people also enjoyed attending the classes and benefited greatly.

Multiple sclerosis

MS (multiple sclerosis) is a disease which affects the central nervous system, a disabling neurological disorder which affects around 100,000 young adults in the UK, between the ages of 20 and 40, affecting more women than men at a ratio of 3:2. It can cause a wide variety of symptoms that vary in severity and duration, ranging from mild and short-lived, to severe and long-lasting.

MS occurs when there is damage to the myelin, the protective coating surrounding all the nerve fibres in the central nervous system, which is made up of the brain and spinal cord. When the myelin becomes damaged it affects the workings of the central nervous system. Damage to nerves that are responsible for movement can result in poor co-ordination, and those responsible for sensation can result in tingling or numbness, but it does not necessarily mean there is anything wrong with the muscles or senses. Putting it in layman's terms, the right messages between the brain, spinal cord or the rest of the body are slower or distorted, and as a result do not get through.

Taking sensible gentle exercise regularly is vitally important to those with the early stages of MS. The healing art of the belly dance stimulates the body's healing process through the nerves and muscles, producing physical and mental changes, which help to maintain muscle control, balance and co-ordination, release tension, and energise.

If you are interested in more information on MS, contact the MS helpline on 0808 800 8000, or email info@mssociety.org.uk

Website: www.mssociety.org.uk

Chronic fatigue

No specific cause for chronic fatigue syndrome or post-viral fatigue, known as ME, or, to be correct, myalgic encephalomyelitis, has yet been found. It has been suggested that it may have developed after an illness resembling a viral or bacterial infection or other medical problems, but evidence to support this theory has recently been dismissed. It is thought to involve both the central nervous system and the immune system. Symptoms include prolonged periods of extreme fatigue, problems in the upper respiratory tract, bladder, bowel and digestive problems, poor circulation, headaches, swollen lymph nodes, muscular aches and pains, and disturbed sleep.

Some people may also develop depression as a result of the illness. The slightest exertion or physical activity can leave a person feeling absolutely exhausted and required to rest for prolonged periods. It is not unknown for some people who have been very seriously affected by this illness to become confined to a wheelchair. Chronic fatigue syndrome can be extremely difficult to diagnose and unfortunately there is no cure. Most people recover in a few weeks, although for some it can be a matter of months, and in severe cases it could be years.

It is important to boost up your immune system and get plenty of rest and at least 7–8 hours' sleep which, I hasten to add, is not always possible. Also, doing regular slow, gentle belly dance movements and the breathing techniques on page 61 will help to play an essential and beneficial role in aiding your recovery by calming down your central nervous system and stimulating your body's healing power.

For further information on chronic fatigue syndrome log on to the website www.meassociation.org.uk. The ME Connect Helpline is available every day from 10am till 12pm; 2pm till 4pm; and 7pm till 9pm on 0844 576 5326.

Fibromyalgia

Fibromyalgia is a term used to describe widespread tenderness, aches and pains that affect the muscles above and below the waist on both sides of the body at a number of points, but do not affect the joints. This is an illness which involves both the body and the mind and can sometimes be triggered by psychological stress or depression, after surgery, or because of a physical trauma.

It has seemed to be more common among women, in the ratio of approximately 9:1, but apparently more men are now being diagnosed with it so these figures may not now be accurate.

It's only in recent years that fibromyalgia has been more understood, as it used to be misdiagnosed as a degenerative disease of the joints. The main symptoms are muscular fatigue, aches and pains, tenderness, stiffness in the muscles, sleep disturbance, tiredness, loss of stamina, and a lack of energy; difficulty in getting up in the mornings because of pain and stiffness; also depression, tension headaches, and having difficulty in carrying out daily tasks, and for some IBS may be a problem. Symptoms and the effects of fibromyalgia can vary considerably from mild to severe and may only last weeks or months at a time but are always liable to return. My doctor told me it could last a lifetime.

Avoid drinking too much coffee, alcohol and tea. Staying physically active is also very important, but avoid high-impact exercises that will jerk your joints, and take up a low-impact gentle exercise like belly dancing which many women are now doing. The movements of the dance will help to increase blood flow and ease muscle spasm of the affected muscles. Muscle spasm is likely to happen due to the limitation of blood flow and oxygen to the affected area.

Gentle exercise stimulates and releases substances called endorphins and encephalin which help to relieve pain, relax muscles, lessen stress mentally and physically. You will also find your sleep patterns improving, which in turn will lessen fatigue.

According to leading researchers in the field of fibromyalgia and chronic fatigue, getting 7 or more hours' sleep a night on a regular basis is one of the most effective ways to eliminate the pain. It is also vitally important for those of you with fibromyalgia to learn to relieve your anxiety and stress by relaxing, which can be done in easy stages.

Only exercise every other day and limit your sessions to begin with to a few minutes, then gradually increase the sessions slowly. Exercise may be a little painful to begin with and you will also feel tired, so don't overdo it, but don't give in. Think positively. Gradually your muscles will become stronger and your fitness levels and general well-being will begin to improve.

Unfortunately there is no quick fix for fibromyalgia and a cure has yet to be discovered, but you can help to lower your levels of pain by doing breathing exercises (on page 61) and by learning to relax. (Refer to page 102 for relaxation techniques.)

If you cannot take medication try a herbal medicinal product called valerian, a root extract which helps to relieve mild anxiety and sleep disturbances.

I have also been diagnosed with fibromyalgia which began at least 4 years ago, so I do know what you are going through. Many women in their fifties believe it started when they came off HRT, and as a result decided to go back on it, although there is no medical evidence to support this. Physically, and mentally, belly dancing has definitely helped me to cope with it, and consultants and my GP have told me that whatever I do I must not stop dancing, which is sometimes easier said than done. But do give it a try and persevere with it.

If you have any of these symptoms, do make an appointment to see your doctor who will explain fibromyalgia to you in more detail and may send you for a blood test. However, a blood test is not usually used to diagnose fibromyalgia, but can rule out other conditions. Then, depending on the results, your GP may recommend a course of medication and/or send you to see a physiotherapist, psychologist or counsellor.

If you want to know more about fibromyalgia you can pick up a leaflet from your doctor's surgery, or you can contact the Fibromyalgia Association UK national helpline on 0844 887 2444,

10am – 4pm Mon–Fri, or email charity@fmauk.org. Visit the website www.fmauk.org or write to Studio 3013, Mile End Mill, 12 Seedhill Rd, Paisley PA1 1JS.

Or contact Arc, committed to curing arthritis, telephone 0870 850 5000; www.arc.org.uk

7. Digestive problems

Life's not just being alive, but being well.
(Epigramma, *Oxford Book of Quotations*)

Ill health is often the result of stress and strain upon the body, mind and spirit. The energy flow becomes blocked, which can result in stomach problems.

Physical exercise is vitally important as it helps to increase the blood flow to the brain and to the muscles, and stimulates the production of natural chemicals called endorphins and encephalin, which have natural pain-relieving properties. This creates a rise in energy levels, which in turn helps to restore physical activity, mobilise and lubricate stiff and aching joints, relax muscle tension, and helps to eliminate anxiety.

I cannot stress enough the importance of taking up a low-impact exercise like belly dancing, whatever your problem, whether it be the early stages of arthritis, endometriosis, multiple sclerosis, fibromyalgia, cancers, chronic fatigue and obesity, dementia, low back pain, IBS and other digestive problems. If you don't exercise, your condition could deteriorate.

For thousands of years tribal communities used the concept of dance to induce some kind of relief from emotional stress anxieties, certain ailments and diseases of the stomach, which to them were believed to be an invasion of demons. These they exorcised through frenzied, contorted and convulsive forms of dance until they collapsed from sheer exhaustion.

IBS (irritable bowel syndrome)

This is a malfunction of the intestine, a very common syndrome thought to be mainly stress-related, although it may be provoked by a gut infection, antibiotics, anti-inflammatory drugs or certain foods, or an excessive consumption of alcohol, which can affect the whole of the digestive system causing irritation, pain, constipation or diarrhoea.

The problem is a functional bowel disorder and not a serious disease of the intestines in the conventional sense. The gut becomes sensitised, which means that the muscles in the wall of the large intestine overreact to nerve impulses in the brain at times of stress.

For some people this condition can be unceasing, and lead to more upsetting symptoms. IBS affects more women than men, and the numerous unpleasant symptoms vary between individuals. A person may feel generally unwell and lethargic, and suffer from one or more of the following symptoms: heartburn and indigestion, intestinal pain which may ease off when the bowels are open, a change in bowel habit, bloating, constipation or diarrhoea, and an urgency to open the bowels first thing in the morning.

Stress is also the main cause of peptic ulcers, but research has shown that smoking, taking aspirin and anti-inflammatory drugs for prolonged periods of time, or an infection of the gut can also increase the risk of peptic ulcers.

For more information, support and advice about IBS, join the IBS network, the UK national charity for patients with irritable bowel syndrome: www.theibsnetwork.org

The IBS network runs a telephone helpline staffed by specialist IBS nurses who will give you professional advice by mail plus much more.

Diverticular disease

This disease, unlike IBS, affects more people in middle age and older. As we age, our internal muscles lose their strength and elasticity, and this, combined with a low-fibre diet, can increase your chance of getting this disorder. Abdominal pain is caused by small pockets that look somewhat like tiny mushrooms protruding from the lining of the large intestine which may become inflamed and infected. A high fibre diet is important in helping to relieve some of these symptoms.

Stomach cancer

This is the second most common cancer after lung cancer, and stress is said to be a contributor. Some experts also believe that long-held resentment can be a factor which eats away at your body and becomes the disease we call cancer.

A bad diet and excess alcohol are also factors. Researchers believe there is a positive link between alcohol consumption and cancers of the digestive system. Alcohol increases the production of stomach acid, which then upsets the balance of acid to mucin (which is the protective lining of the stomach walls). When this protective lining becomes damaged, inflammation and ulcers in the intestine flare up. This causes flatulence, which can be very uncomfortable and for some painful. IBS and digestive problems can be relieved by changing your eating habits and de-stressing, by doing breathing exercises, relaxation, and concentrating on belly dance movements of the abdomen and pelvic region which will calm down your central nervous system and activate the free flow of energy.

Over the years women of all ages with various forms of cancer have come along to my belly dance classes, some after surgery and others while in remission, and got immense benefits from doing the belly dance movements. They described belly dancing as an holistic activity which empowered them and boosted their energy levels. Some made full recoveries, but sadly others didn't.

8. Endometriosis

Endometriosis is a painful disease of the pelvic organs that affects women in their reproductive years, due to the presence of endometrium which is normally confined to the mucous membrane lining the cavity of the uterus. When found in other parts of the pelvic cavity such as on the ovaries and fallopian tubes, localised pain occurs, causing severe period pains and back pain. According to infertility specialists, endometriosis is the cause of infertility in many women, but little is known about what causes endometriosis.

Getting in touch with one's sexuality and femininity through the belly dance can be a significant factor in helping to reduce the symptoms.

Belly dancing and breathing techniques have helped numerous women with the early stages of endometriosis, pre-menstrual tension, menstrual and menopausal problems, through the movements that concentrate on the abdominal and pelvic region as they increase the production of endorphins and reduce oestrogen levels, having a positive effect on the central nervous system. Some women told me that they became addicted to belly dancing because of the relief they gained.

Success story

A woman contacted me after having heard me on a radio programme saying that belly dancing was an excellent form of exercise for those with the early stages of endometriosis and that it may even help some women to conceive. She told me she had the early stages of endometriosis and desperately wanted a baby and had been trying to conceive for years. After her first session, I gave her a list of belly dance movements and some sexercises to do which she promised to practise at home. She continued to come to class for at least a year, then suddenly stopped coming.

Eighteen months later I got a lovely letter from her saying that she had had a baby girl several months before and was ecstatic. She was convinced that if she hadn't come along to my belly dancing classes she would never have become pregnant – plus she sent me a very big thank-you.

Endometriosis Free Helpline: 0808 808 2227 or email enquiries@endometriosis-uk.org

9. The heart

The importance of a healthy heart

The heart in its smallness sustains its owner.
Many are the small things that are worthy of respect.
– The twentieth instruction
(*The Little Book of Egyptian Wisdom* compiled by Naomi Ozaniec)

Heart disease is the biggest killer in the Western world and affects people of all ages and backgrounds, and sadly most of these deaths could have been prevented. A heart attack can be attributed to a family history of heart disease, but most commonly is caused by smoking, drinking too much alcohol, lack of exercise, high blood pressure, high cholesterol levels and obesity. Having more than one of these factors is cause for concern. Our heart is made up mainly of muscle, which rhythmically contracts and relaxes as it pumps blood and oxygen around our body and eliminates waste matter from tissue and organs.

In our lifetime, our heart will beat approximately three million times and pump 9 litres of blood around our body each day.

Coronary arteries are tubes which carry blood to the heart and if the arteries fur up, it increases the chances of them becoming blocked, which makes a person vulnerable to a heart attack. High cholesterol levels are known to have a direct effect on the heart.

As cholesterol levels rise, there is a greater risk of furred-up arteries. Obesity and diabetes in women is also associated with the furring-up of the arteries more than in men.

Poor blood circulation affects our body and our organs in numerous ways because it prevents the blood flow from efficiently reaching our vital organs and cells. Poor circulation also affects our brain cells, causing memory loss and other problems such as headaches, migraines and dizziness.

However, research evidence suggests that for some people, stress may contribute towards heart disease. There is growing evidence that stress is also linked to coronary heart disease, but is not one of the main risk factors.

The highest risk factor is smoking which has disastrous consequences on your heart, causing coronary heart disease. Smoking also contributes to other high-risk illnesses such as cancer of the lungs, mouth and larynx and other parts of the body such as the gut, bladder and kidneys. Smoking also causes emphysema and chronic bronchitis.

Every time you take a puff of a cigarette you inhale numerous poisonous chemicals, including carbon monoxide and nicotine. Carbon monoxide affects the levels of oxygen the blood carries around your body by reducing the amount of oxygen the blood can carry. Nicotine produces adrenalin which stimulates your body, making your heart beat much quicker than normal, which raises your blood pressure and stresses the heart by making it work harder.

Risk factors for coronary disease can be prevented by cutting down on the amount of alcohol you drink, eating less fatty foods and ignoring junk food. Eat sensibly and include plenty of vegetables and fruit in your diet, as they contain antioxidants which could prevent your arteries furring up. Also include pasta, beans, rice, pulses and potatoes in your diet, and cut down your intake of sugar and salt and control your blood sugar levels. If you make a determined effort to lower your cholesterol you will help reduce your risk of heart disease.

Exercising regularly is vitally important in helping to improve and maintain a healthy cardiovascular system. So take up a low-impact physical activity such as belly dancing which is an ideal exercise if you are unfit. The gentle belly dance movements and abdominal exercises such as tummy rolls, flutters and rib cage movements will work those core muscles, increasing and improving your circulation and muscle tone which includes your heart.

Exercising regularly will strengthen your heart muscles, help to keep your weight down, calm and stimulate your mind, boost your body's vitality, and tone up your flabby belly which will help to get rid of that belly flab (that's the fat that hangs down over the tummy, yuck). Breathing correctly will also lower your heart rate and help to tone up those flabby tummies. (Refer to page 61 for breathing techniques).

Swimming and walking are also very good types of low-impact exercise. However, before starting your exercise regime consult your GP or physician who will consider your health and fitness levels and advise you on how much exercise you should do. Whatever exercise regime you choose, remember to always start with some gentle warm-ups to get your blood circulating – not stretching exercises as you need to warm up before doing those.

If you have any concerns about these health issues, contact your GP or call Heart Matters on 0300 330 3311 or email heart-matters@bhs.org.uk

10. Obesity or ESA morbidly obese

Eat to live. Don't live to eat.
(Benjamin Franklin)

Obese and morbidly obese people are putting their lives in

jeopardy on a daily basis, exposing themselves to many serious and life-threatening health issues such as Type 2 diabetes, a major health problem which affects the body's ability to process sugar, which can lead to many life-threatening diseases. Obesity has become a very worrying health problem in Western society as it has now reached epidemic proportions among adults of both sexes. Researchers claim that over three million people now suffer from the condition in the UK and that is really frightening. It is also becoming a great financial strain on the National Health Service (NHS) as it is costing billions of pounds to treat. Even more worrying is the growing trend of obesity in children, who are being put at great risk. Children in the UK are said to be the fattest and most unhealthy in Europe. Research suggests it's more than likely they are being put at risk by a family member who is also obese.

There is a great concern about the unhealthy eating habits of children which can lead to health problems in adulthood, putting them in great danger of being exposed to life-threatening illnesses; as a result they will more than likely die before their parents. As a parent you need to be responsible and recognise that too much fat and sugar in the body plus a lack of physical activity can damage internal organs and seriously affect your children's health.

For some people obesity is genetic, or due to a specific drug, illness or a psychological problem, but for the majority it is a result of gluttony, sedentary lifestyles and downright laziness, an illness that could be prevented if you looked after yourself and exercised regularly to increase your body's energy. Eat sensibly by avoiding fatty foods which have high levels of saturated fat, sugars and salt. You can start helping yourself by cutting down on your intake of sugar, and fatty foods such as chips, burgers and greasy fry-ups. Avoid those tempting cream cakes, sweets, chocolates, alcohol and bottles of fizzy drinks which have a very frightening high-sugar content that causes acid erosion and tooth decay, a serious problem which is now affecting thousands of children. Also check cereals, sausages and other meat products before purchasing as some may also contain sugar and molasses. It's a fallacy that you need sugar to give you energy; I have been intolerant to sugar since birth but it hasn't affected my energy levels.

Don't overeat, gobble down your food or have irregular meals. Adopting bad eating habits, such as sitting in front of the television with the meal on your lap, doesn't help, as it can cause digestive problems.

Personal problems such as stress, tension and depression, low self-esteem, boredom, unhappiness, negativity and a lack of exercise can lead to comfort eating, and are problems that urgently need to be addressed to prevent the onset of obesity, and the life-threatening health issues that may arise from obesity.

Although it is fair to say that people who are not obese can suffer from the health problems that I have mentioned, obese people are more at risk because obesity is fraught with numerous serious related health issues such as cardiovascular disease (affecting the heart), high blood pressure and cholesterol levels, secondary diabetes, difficulty in breathing and some types of cancer, heartburn, strokes, blindness and loss of limbs. Obesity causes lack of mobility which causes problems such as not being able to climb stairs, get out of your bed, or in and out of your chair, dress yourself and walk any reasonable distance without difficulty and becoming breathless. Obesity also causes back pain and physical damage to hip and knee joints, which may eventually have to be replaced by artificial joints.

At some time or other we all make unhealthy choices and make wrong decisions, especially under pressure, and I suppose we can put a little of the blame for that on modern society. So where do you start? How can you help yourself and your family to adopt a healthier regime? Well, first you will need an enormous amount of determination, positive-ness, and also the help and support of your family.

Make a positive attempt now to change your lifestyle and improve your diet. Substitute those unhealthy drinks for two or three glasses of water, fruit juice or a cup of tea, without milk or sugar. Prepare and eat plenty of fresh wholesome foods which include vegetables and fruit, fish, chicken, lean meats, rice and pasta. (I can already hear the moans and someone saying "I don't like vegetables, I don't cook and I won't cook – I hate cooking!") Yes, shopping for wholesome food and cooking a meal will take up some of your time, but cooking can be great fun and rewarding, especially if you can involve your children.

Sitting down to a home-cooked meal all together at the table is something both you and your family will greatly benefit from, by improving your general health and well-being and by enjoying the social interaction within your family group.

I do believe that children from a young age should be taught cooking and nutrition in schools to encourage a healthier lifestyle.

Take up an activity, one that the whole family can participate in. A low-impact exercise like swimming, walking or belly dancing will help your cardiovascular and respiratory system, tone your muscles and strengthen the muscles which surround and support your internal organs, firm up your flabby tummy, improve your mobility and flexibility, raise your self-esteem, and relieve tension and depression.

Do not go running, jogging, or jump up and down, as such exercises will put more stress and strain on your hip, knee and ankle joints which may cause long-term damage. Also wear a good support bra when exercising or dancing.

Young children also love belly dancing. I have groups of children who come along regularly to my classes with their mums. It's lovely to see mums and their children doing something special together and enjoying it.

People have the impression that if you take up belly dancing you will have to show your belly. Well, let me reassure you, you don't. I don't.

Most importantly, don't give in. I know it won't be easy and there will be numerous times when you will be tempted to say "To hell with all of this!", go back to your old habits and plonk yourself down in front of the telly with a meal on your lap which you have taken straight from the freezer and put into a microwave, plus a litre of fizzy drink or a few pints of beer to wash it all down with.

Please persevere. When you have succeeded you will be so proud of yourself and your family, and so will your friends. There is a lot of help out there for you, but at the end of the day you and you alone are responsible for the majority of your obesity problems. So be aware of what food and drink you are putting into your shopping trolley. Do you really want to spend the rest of your precious life with the kind of serious and debilitating life-threatening health problems I have mentioned? Or worse still, seriously damage the health of your child? Make a determined effort to start now, today, and why not? My granddad always said to me, "Never put off anything until tomorrow that you can do today."

Contact your GP for advice; he or she will refer you to your local health and well-being centres and slimming clubs.

You can also become a supporter of Change4Life, supported by the Department of Health, who have launched a campaign which sets out to tackle serious health issues. Helpline: 0300 123 3434 or go to www.nhs.uk/change4life and click onto 'partners and supporters'.

11. Diet

You are what you eat. Tell me what you eat and I'll tell you what you are.
(*Physiologie du Gout*, 1825)

Personally I do not believe that dieting is actually good for you. It cannot be beneficial to your health to go on a crash diet because you're going on holiday or to a special event, then start to pile on the pounds again. But adopting a healthy diet, i.e. eating sensibly on a daily basis, can without a doubt completely turn your life around. Not only will you lose weight, but you will also feel less sluggish, more energetic and happier in yourself. A healthy activity such as belly dancing combined with a healthy diet is extremely important and both should complement each other to get the full benefits of them together. There is a wealth of material already written about diets and healthy eating and self-help groups such as Weight Watchers; some may work and others not. However, eating sensibly is really a matter of common sense, but for many this is not an easy option, as shoppers are presented with an abundance of tempting pre-packed foods, convenience foods, and over-refined foods which are high in calories and fat, low in nutrients and fibre. These foods seriously add on the pounds and cause digestive problems, lower the immune system, cause vitamin deficiencies and mineral imbalances, hormonal imbalance and depression. Even if you are on a special medically prescribed diet, it is worth keeping in mind the fundamental structure of a well-balanced diet. You can achieve a wise pattern of eating by following a few simple guidelines; it's not rocket science. Cut down on foods which contain high levels of animal fats, stodgy foods, fried foods, refined sugar and starch, and avoid drinking large amounts of liquids while eating.

A healthy balanced diet should include a daily intake of fresh fruit and vegetables, which, when eaten raw, supply various kinds of fibre, health-giving vitamins and minerals. Cream-free milk, or soya milk, eggs, yogurt, lean meat, fish, poultry and nuts will provide the necessary amount of protein and calcium.

Wholegrain products which contain vitamin D, like bran, whole wheat cereals, wholemeal bread and flour, will supply an adequate amount of natural fibre in your diet, and I stress again, drink plenty of fluids, including at least a couple of glasses of water a day, fruit juices and tea; try some green tea instead of those sugary fizzy drinks. Your body needs fluids as they are vitally important in helping to prevent dehydration and maintain a healthy body.

The benefits of green tea have been researched for many decades and it has now been hailed as a miracle. It's found to have powerful antioxidants, removes free radicals, and is very beneficial in helping to protect your health in many ways. Combined with a healthy diet and gentle exercise it can help to keep the heart healthy by lowering cholesterol and the risk of heart disease, controlling blood pressure problems and cutting the risk of having a stroke. It's also beneficial to those of you with diabetes. It's also believed to help to prevent weight gain and help those of you who are obese by suppressing the appetite.

Researchers also have found that green tea lowers the risk of cancer and could help to ward off dementia. It cuts out bad breath and improves oral health.

When you purchase your green tea try to get the organic or pure type which is available from most supermarkets; better still, if possible get the loose tea leaves – it's said they are more beneficial.

When introduced to some foods it's more than likely you or your children will look at them and say, "I don't like that." How do you know you don't like it until you've tasted it? Surely it's a better option than ill health and having to take medication.

To detoxify, start your day by drinking a small glass of warm water with a teaspoonful of organic apple cider vinegar which has many health benefits as it contributes to healthier blood vessels and arteries. Apple cider vinegar has a phenomenal amount of potassium and malic acid which is very beneficial. You could also add a spoonful of good-quality honey to the vinegar and water which should be warm enough to melt the honey.

Purchase your local honey, or Manuka honey produced in New Zealand which is the best honey you can buy, but it is very expensive. Apparently if you suffer from hay fever your local honey is a more effective treatment. Honey is also good for healing wounds.

Note: To protect the enamel on your teeth it's advisable to drink through a straw to avoid the acid in the vinegar damaging your teeth.

For more tips on vinegar for health and personal care, read *Vinegar: 1001 Practical Uses* by Margaret Briggs. It's a fascinating, inexpensive little book.

You can become a supporter of Change4Life which is supported by the Department of Health, who have launched a campaign which sets out to tackle serious health issues. Their helpline is 0300 123 3434 or go to www.nhs.uk/change4life and click onto 'partners and supporters'.

In the Middle East, North Africa and in some European countries women are more curvaceous and rounded and have a more positive attitude about themselves. When I was in the Middle East men told me that they liked their women big and would get 300 or more camels for their wives. With a grin they offered only three camels for me.

12. Antioxidants and free radicals

The terms antioxidants and free radicals are often used these days and it may help to understand what they are. Free radicals are described as organic molecules which are responsible for causing damage to healthy tissue and believed to cause some diseases. Antioxidants are found in vitamins E and C and beta carotenes, which interact with free radicals and help to maintain a healthy body by boosting our immune system and preventing illnesses such as cancer, premature ageing and other diseases.

If you want to avoid ill health and maintain a healthy body

and mind, you must eat sensibly and help your body to get rid of the free radicals by including the following in your diet: cabbage, broccoli and other leafy green vegetables, and green peppers, sweet potatoes, beans, nuts, fish oils, whole grains, oranges, lemons, fruit juices, kiwi fruit, strawberries and blueberries.

0800 077 3564 www.feelkarma.com

13. Skeletal problems

The skeletal system and back pain

Prevention is better than cure.
(Early 17th century)

Back pain is a very common problem, generally due to improper use of the spine. Lack of spinal mobilisation constricts the joints, which as a result fail to function properly, causing stiffness, discomfort, aches and pains in varying degrees. The spinal column consists of 24 segments of bone, which are stacked on top of one another. The lumbar spine or lower back is made up of five vertebrae, twelve make up the thorax (the chest area of the spine) and seven make up the neck.

Like all other joints, muscles control their movements. These muscles can become tired, distort and twist, which sometimes pulls the spine out of alignment. Belly dance movements are based on the natural structure of the body and help to move the body as it is designed to move, which eliminates stress on the joints and muscles. The gentle rhythmic belly dance movements such as hip rotations, pelvic tilts, pelvic rolls and hip pushes will help to mobilise the spine, allow self-lubrication and improved blood circulation, ease muscle spasms, stiffness, and relieve pain. The ability to move freely is vitally important to our overall health and well-being.

The spine in the lower back and the pelvic floor muscles play a pivotal role in protecting the back. Physiotherapists may also show you some deep breathing techniques which will help to relieve your back pain.

Strain can be put on the spine as a result of being overweight, injury or poor posture, carrying heavy bags on one's shoulder or a child on the hip which causes you to lean over to one side, daily activities such as housework and gardening, prolonged sitting and using seating that does not support the curvature of the spine effectively. Mattresses that do not support the back adequately, lifting and carrying something incorrectly (which does not have to be a heavy item), or too much assertive exercise can also cause problems. Poor posture is the cause of many back complaints. Pot bellies and beer bellies also cause back problems. To alleviate your back problem get rid of that belly and work those 'abs' (abdominal muscles), and strengthen those core muscles which support your spine. Belly dancing is an excellent core workout combined with specific breathing techniques. If you do the abdominal and pelvic exercises on a regular basis they will help to strengthen the muscles in your back. Numerous women with low back problems tell me how much their back problem has improved or completely disappeared since taking up belly dancing. Mr Mushtaque Ishaque, a spinal surgeon at the Royal Orthopaedic Hospital and BMI Priory Hospital in Birmingham, UK, says (quoted from the *Daily Mail*): "Those who are suffering from back pain are taught to target the core muscles. These are the transverse abdominus, the muscle which runs between the ribs and the pelvis, and the multifidus (next to the spine in the lower back) and the pelvic floor muscles. Together, they play a pivotal role in protecting the back."

To improve your posture all you have to do is assume the starting position. Raise your rib cage, drop your shoulders and relax your knees; if you have done this correctly then your spine will be naturally aligned. As I have already mentioned, *don't pull your shoulders back* as many experts will tell you to do, as it puts a strain on your upper back and is also a very uncomfortable and an un-relaxed position to hold.

Correct seating is not always available, especially in a working environment. If you slump when sitting, it causes the back to twist, which is bad for the joints, muscles and ligaments and affects your blood circulation. Ideally, you should sit in a chair that gives you comfortable support up to the back of your head. Your lower back should be against the back of the chair, your bottom at the same level as your knees, or slightly higher, and both feet flat on the floor.

There is nothing worse than trying to sleep on an uncomfortable mattress, especially if you have a back problem. There are many opinions and confusion as to what type of mattress is best. When purchasing a bed your weight and height should be taken into consideration and also your age. What was comfortable for you at 35 won't be comfortable at 75. A good bed should comfortably take your weight and prevent your spine from lapsing into an extreme posture by firmly supporting the healthy curvature of the spine. If you already suffer from a back problem, a soft or sagging mattress may cause the spine to sag and bring on pain whether you lie on your back, side or front.

Many back sufferers have been encouraged to purchase, at great expense, the latest super-orthopaedic bed which they then find impossible to sleep on. It is generally accepted that the stiffer the spine, the more difficult it is to adapt to a very hard bed. A healthy elastic spine needs more support while sleeping, therefore a firmer mattress is advisable.

People with back pain sometimes believe that bed rest will relieve their pain. However, while in an acute stage with muscle spasm this can be a good thing, it is advisable to seek treatment before the back becomes stiff. Lack of movement can sometimes lead to the back freezing up. But by gently doing the belly dance movements one can regain mobility.

Back pain is diagnosed as either chronic or acute. Chronic

pain is a persistent, prolonged ache that eventually becomes a very severe pain which will not ease until treated. Acute pain will, more often than not, eventually ease of its own accord in a few days or weeks.

For help and advice, contact the Back Care Charity www.backcare.org.uk. You can also call the Sleep Council Helpline: 0845 058 4595 and 01756 791089, or go to www.sleep-council.com. The 'Bed Buyer's Guide' is free from the Sleep Council.

14. Learners' general complaints

Movement is a blessing.
(Arabic, anonymous)

Sciatica

Sciatica is the result of pressure on a nerve at the base of the spine, which may be a result of lifting or twisting awkwardly. The pain may go from the buttocks to the calf and foot of one leg, making the leg and foot feel weak and numb. Manipulative practitioners or physiotherapists will re-align your spine and treat any pain and discomforts relating to the back, and advise you on whether to use a heat pad or ice pack. A painful or aching knee can also be a consequence of a back problem.

Slipped disc

The term 'slipped disc' is a misconception. Movement does not dislodge the discs, which sit firmly between two vertebrae acting as a buffer and protector. Each disc has a pulpy nucleus surrounded by a granular hard ring. What happens is that the ring splits under stress or strain and the nucleus leaks into the vertebral cavity and presses on the nerves. This is a very painful problem, but it can be remedied by gentle manipulation performed by a medical or manipulative practitioner.

Treatments will help to re-align your spine and treat any other discomfort or pain relating to your back. Once this has been treated successfully, you should be able to continue with some gentle belly dance movements.

Frozen shoulder

'Frozen shoulder' is a fairly common affliction of the shoulder joint which becomes progressively restricted in movement and increasingly painful and stiff. Severe cases can take more than two years to resolve.

Treatment will help restore some space within the joint so that the head of the humerus, the long bone in the arm which extends from the shoulder to the elbow, has room to manoeuvre. This problem is not easily treatable, so exercise should be taken with caution. For some sufferers surgery may be the only option, so do seek advice from a practitioner who will recommend a programme of corrective treatment and exercise. As long as pain persists it is not advisable to do any elevation of the arms or shoulder shimmies, but you will be able to do many other belly dance movements in class.

Clicking

When dancing, many students become anxious if they experience a clicking sound in their hips and knees. This is caused by bubbles of synovial fluid popping like a release of air from a vacuum. Sometimes tendons move and click over the bone surface, but this is nothing to worry about. Many of us have experienced an example of this 'clicking' when we have pulled our fingers. Remedy – a good massage.

Note: Pain is a warning of the body's dysfunction due to either emotional distress, disease or injury and should not be ignored.

Knee problems

The patella (knee cap) and the knee joint can be affected by a number of problems such as a torn cartilage, sprained ligaments or strained muscle due to a fall or a sports injury, arthritis or bursitis, and one type known as housemaid's knee. Soft tissue damage causes inflammation and, as a consequence, tenderness, swelling and bruising occur, which results in stiffness and lack of mobility. Knee strain can also be caused by a torn cartilage due to a sudden twist of the knee or by turning in the foot. Many learners tend to turn their foot inwards, which twists in the knee when stepping forward or when placing the foot forward with the heel raised. This is something I always discourage by bringing it to the attention of learners as the majority of them are not aware that they do it, and thankfully for some learners it can be rectified.

Bending the knees too much or dancing with knees bent affects the line of gravity from falling correctly. The knees should only be flexed slightly, bent no more than 5 degrees, and feet should be held firmly to the floor.

Being overweight puts a tremendous amount of stress on your knees and as a result they are made to work much harder, so it's important you lose weight to help improve your mobility; otherwise you may end up having to have knee replacements. Moving your knees to and fro rapidly will also damage your knees; many teachers will instruct you to move your knees in this way while shimmying on the spot. To avoid damage to your knees they should be relaxed and held steady while shimmying.

Belly dance movements, particularly the hip shimmy and pelvic tilts with alternative contractions, will exercise the gluteus (the large muscles in your bottom) which will help to reduce stiffness and strengthen the thigh muscles, which will stabilise the knees and help to improve your mobility. If your 'glutes' are weak, it can affect your hips and knees. Dr Pippa Bennett, a musculo-skeletal physician, says (quoted from a UK national newspaper): "Weak glutes can cause the knee to fall inwards when walking, causing wear on the inner side of the knee joint.

Arthritis can then develop. Weak bottom muscles can also cause the weight of the body to bear down excessively on the hips, causing osteoarthritis."

If you have had a knee problem your practitioner will advise you when to start exercising or dancing.

15. Dyspraxia – a neurological disorder of motor co-ordination

Dyspraxia, a term derived from a Greek word meaning 'movement process', is described as a very complex neurological disorder, a variable condition that manifests itself in many different ways in people of various ages. Symptoms vary and may include poor balance, co-ordination, perceptual problems, difficulty in planning motor tasks, and problems with spatial awareness.

Unfortunately this is a problem that is too easy to dismiss through ignorance, with some dance and fitness teachers believing the learner is just clumsy or thick. We are all aware that lack of ability to do something correctly can cause us frustration and undue stress.

Dyspraxia is described as a variable symptom, not a condition, and is often divided into two different types: verbal dyspraxia known as apraxia of speech, and dyspraxia known as development co-ordination disorder which is apparent from birth or early age.

Co-ordination disorder was not recognised as a symptom when today's elderly were young, but today it is recognised at an early age. Prognosis greatly varies and there are numerous confusing terms used to describe dyspraxia.

Many senior learners have told me of their frustration and that they have walked out of a class feeling upset because they were ignored and left to struggle with the movements. If you have poor co-ordination and other related problems you need a teacher who is patient and understanding, and will not dismiss your difficulties. It may have taken you a lot of courage to join a class, so don't give in. Have a word with the teacher and explain your difficulties. If your problem is ignored and you find yourself still struggling, it would be advisable to find another teacher.

Approved dyspraxia helpline: 01462 454 986

16. Freedom of movement

Exercise – you don't have time not to.
(Unknown source)

Movement is the ability to move freely with strength and agility. Lack of exercise prevents the joints from carrying out their full range of movement, which eventually leads to a deterioration of the joints, causing further problems of a more serious nature.

Joints that are attached to muscles by tendons and ligaments move the bones of the skeleton. The bone ends are protected by articular cartilage. A capsule that has a synovial membrane lining exudes a clear, lubricating, nourishing fluid surrounding the joint. Synovial joints are self-lubricating as they produce their own fluid, but the synovial fluid can only be produced if there is movement between the two bones.

Movement is extremely important, because it helps to stimulate the synovial membrane to function properly between two articulating surfaces. If there is no movement, the fluid will not be produced and the joints will become dry and stiff, causing arthritis. The gentle movements of the belly dance are an ideal form of exercise because belly dance movements are a natural and effective way of assisting your body to move in the way it is designed to move. Arthritis is a common condition that varies from a mild ache to extreme pain and affects more women than men. It's often a condition that is associated with old age but that is not necessarily so. It may also be a hereditary condition for some.

Occasionally some learners complain of a crunching sensation in their hips when dancing; this could be an early sign of arthritis and shouldn't be ignored. So seek medical advice as soon as possible.

Rheumatoid arthritis is a severe type of arthritis, a chronic and extremely painful disease. The membranes of the joints become swollen, stiff, lose their mobility and become deformed.

Osteoarthritis is a very painful degenerative joint disease that commonly affects the hips, knees or fingers; it occurs when the protective layer of cartilage that covers the surface of the joint deteriorates, causing pain and impaired mobility of the affected joint which can worsen as one gets older and disrupt one's normal daily activities. You must keep mobile and active even if the pain is unbearable, which I know is the last thing one wants to do when in pain, but it is a necessary evil. Movement is necessary to help stimulate the synovial fluid and improve the flow of blood to the affected joint. If you don't make an attempt to exercise, your condition will worsen and become even more painful.

If you have the early or advanced stages of arthritis, rheumatoid arthritis or osteoarthritis, cut out high-impact exercise – that's a definite no. No running, jogging or jumping over hurdles! Stick to low-impact exercise, like belly dancing. Learners with the early stages of the above conditions have greatly benefited both physically and psychologically from doing belly dancing on a regular basis. If you smoke make a determined effort to stop; smoking has a detrimental effect on the bones and joints and health in general. Improve your diet and regulate your alcohol intake.

If you have osteoarthritis your doctor will advise you on a course of treatment or refer you to see an orthopaedic consultant who may recommend that you have a joint replacement.

Muriel, a delightful learner when in her seventies, attended one of my summer schools in the 1980s. She suffered from arthritis, and constantly needed the support of her walking stick. Four days into the course she became so excited, because for the first time in years she could walk without the aid of her walking stick. The reason was that while learning the dance movements, her posture, balance, co-ordination and flexibility had dramatically improved, easing much discomfort and pain. At the end of the week, to our astonishment, she actually abseiled down the side of the Sheffield University building! What a fantastic woman!

17. Osteoporosis

One in two females over the age of 50 in the UK will be diagnosed with osteoporosis, a condition which increases with age, and becomes more progressive when one reaches the menopause, swiftly beginning to accelerate when we reach the age of 75 or over.

Bone loss happens when the bones begin to thin and weaken, which makes them prone to fractures. Healthy bones are made up of a thick outer shell and a strong inner mesh which is described as looking similar to a honeycomb.

Bones are continuously being reproduced by two types of cells, one that makes new bone, and the other which breaks down the old bone – a process that stays steady until about the age of 35.

Staying active and exercising sensibly and regularly during adolescence will help to maintain healthy bones, and also help to prevent loss of height in our old age. You can reduce the risk of osteoporosis by avoiding high-impact exercises and taking up belly dancing, a non-impact, weight-bearing exercise, as the movements of the dance will support the weight of your body without stress or strain, help to strengthen the bones, and improve muscle tone and balance. Help yourself and avoid smoking, limit your intake of alcohol, and eat your green vegetables and fresh fruit which are rich in calcium.

Your doctor will probably send you for a scan which will measure your bone density. He or she may then prescribe medication to help build bone density, and recommend you to a physiotherapist.

National Osteoporosis Society Helpline: 0845 450 0230 or 01761 472721, open Monday to Friday, 9am till 5pm, excluding bank holidays. Overseas callers: +44 1761 472721. Website: www.nos.org.uk

Rheumatoid Arthritis Helpline: 0808 800 4050, Monday to Friday, 10am till 4pm. Or go to www.arthritiscare.org.uk

Manipulative therapists

Many doctors, chiropractors, osteopaths and physiotherapists are now aware of the health benefits of belly dance, and may even recommend that you attend a class. I am often asked, "What is the difference between a chiropractor, an osteopath, and a physiotherapist?"

Chiropractic is a method of treating diseases by concentrating on manipulation of the skeletal-muscular system of the body. In order to rehabilitate the normal nervous system function, chiropractors adjust the spinal column manually, which may be dysfunctional or partially misaligned.

Osteopathy is the theory of disease and a system of treatment or healing, which mainly consists of massage and manipulation to keep the body in structural balance, so it can heal itself. The practice is based on the supposition that deformation, notably of subsequent interference with blood vessels and nerves, is believed to be the cause of most diseases.

Physiotherapy is the treatment of diseases by remedies involving therapeutic use of physical methods such as massage, remedial exercise, ultraviolet or infrared rays and fresh air.

Acupuncture is a traditional Chinese complementary and alternative medicine involving the penetration of needles which are used to stimulate specific acupuncture points; this corrects imbalances in the flow of *gi* through channels called meridians. Acupuncture is used to treat a range of conditions, especially for pain relief.

18. A woman's cycle

This sacred dance

There is wisdom in the body
That is older than clocks and calendars.
(Hazrat Khan)

This sacred dance, the oldest since civilisation, was a profound and powerful means through which women celebrated their sexual energy, fertility and motherhood, and harmonised with the universe. In ancient times there was no doubt women's monthly cycles harmonised with the lunar cycle, and it is believed that lunar calendars from Upper Palaeolithic times had been used as obstetric calendars.

The moon's patterns divide into four distinct phases: new, waxing, full, and waning moon; each phase lasting approximately 7 days. Hence the belief in matriarchal times that women's monthly cycles followed the same duration as the moon's cycle. Once a month mainly at night, excluding men, groups of women gathered together when menstruating to celebrate the power of fertility through this sacred dance.

There are numerous reasons for disturbances and discomforts during the menstrual cycle, and persistent problems should be medically checked. However, numerous women have found that the belly-dancing movements have greatly helped to alleviate many discomforts and pain, and tell me they have actually become addicted to the belly dance for those reasons.

19. Pregnancy, childbirth and the belly dance

The same stream of life that runs through my veins night and day runs through the world and dances in rhythmic measure.

It is the same life that shoots in joy through the dust of the earth in numberless waves of grass and breaks into tumultuous waves of leaves and flowers.

It is the same life that is rocked in the ocean – cradle of birth and of death, in ebb and flow.

I feel my limbs are made glorious by the touch of this world of life. And my pride is from the life throb of ages dancing in my blood this moment.

– Rabindranath Tagore, *Gitanjali*, 1xix

(Sheila Kitzinger, *The Experience of Childbirth*, 1962)

The birth dance, which originated in pre-biblical times, facilitated birthing and celebrated motherhood. Armen Ohanian, a Persian dancer from the 19th century, wrote in her book *The Dancer of Shamakha* (now out of print): "Such is the veneration of motherhood there are countries and tribes whose binding oath is sworn upon the stomach because it is from this that the sacred cup of humanity has issued."

It was and still is a popular custom in some parts of Egypt for a bride and groom to be pictured with their hands resting on a belly dancer's stomach, a derivation of sacred dances practised in fertility cults. The Hawaiian childbirth preparations known as the *hula* or *ohela*, which are no longer practised, involved movements of the abdomen and pelvic area. Maori women also practised similar movements up until the mid-1930s, and in Central Africa the birth of a child celebrated the transmission of life.

According to Farob Firdoz, a dancer from Bahrain off the coast of Saudi Arabia, the belly dance has its roots in the birth dance. She claimed to have witnessed such rituals in less Westernised parts of her country. During birth rituals, which were considered sacred to women, from which the men were barred. When the mother-to-be was about to give birth the women of the community gathered around the pallet or birthing stool, lamenting and echoing her cries, while rolling their hips and abdomen in earthy circular motions, rocking their pelvises to and fro in an exaggerated manner and shaking their hips.

The aim was to encourage the woman in labour to concentrate on her pelvic region and abdomen, and facilitate the birth by reducing pain during contractions of the womb. This procedure also encouraged the mother-to-be to move with instead of against her contractions, thereby assisting nature instead of fighting against it. After the birth the women expressed their joy through the dance, exaggerating the movements which had assisted the mother during her labour.

Morocco, a dancer from New York, told me she also had an experience similar to that of Farob Firdoz. After befriending a Saudi Arabian woman while on her travels, she was invited to take part in a Berber tribal ceremony, a ceremony very reminiscent of ancient times. In order to be permitted to attend the event she had to take on the role of a mute serving girl of her benefactor. While the men waited outside the tent, the women inside the tent prepared for the birth, which began by digging a hole out of the ground for the mother-to-be to squat over while giving birth.

As labour commenced, her family and friends gathered around her, mimicking her cries as they rippled and rolled their bellies, circled and swayed their hips, and made exaggerated pelvic movements to the rhythmic beat of the drums in an effort to encourage the woman to participate actively during labour and the actual birth.

Until birthing bricks and birthing stools were introduced,

women squatted on the ground or in a hole dug out of the ground. Eventually bricks or stones were placed under each foot of the mother-to-be. As an alternative, women either squatted or knelt on a wooden seat, which had a hole cut out of the centre, large enough for the baby to drop through. The *mshnt*, a kind of birthing chair made of bricks, is believed to have been in use before 2500 BC. This particular chair was eventually replaced by a wooden structure, but when is not known.

Although none of these chairs have survived, it is assumed they were of similar design to those used by the Fallaheen, Egyptian peasant farmers.

Most women gave birth unaided, but on some occasions a midwife, who usually brought along her own birthing stool, attended. During the final stages of labour the midwife squatted in front of the mother-to-be, ready to assist if and when necessary. Unfortunately childbirth all too often resulted in tragedy due to difficult and traumatic births.

There is little information or evidence from ancient Egypt of women's roles in childbirth rites, apart from that collated and pieced together from surveying depictions on temple walls and carvings, plus extracts from myths and stories. That is, apart from that detailed in the Westcar Papyrus, which tells us of Reddjedt's labour and the birth of her triplets.

During her labour the goddess Nephathys supported her from behind and assisted her. The goddess Isis stood before her and the goddess Hekat used her magic to hasten the birth. It is also said that the goddess Hathor assisted at a royal birth, in birth houses such as the one at Phillea temple. Reliefs tell the story of birth and rebirth, and in the temple of Kom Ombo the goddess Isis is seen sitting in the birthing position.

(Source: Barbara Watterson, *Women in Ancient Egypt*, Alan Sutton Publishing, US)

Ritual birth dances survived for thousands of years, but sadly they are now dying out, mainly due to Western society's influences and attitudes.

In societies today the movements of the belly dance are seen as nothing more than a series of amusing and sexually titillating gyrations, instead of a beautiful ancient art form and a natural form of exercise that has aided women in childbirth for thousands of years. This attitude, born out of ignorance, has affected generations of Berber and Bedouin mothers-to-be of the Sahara Desert, who in the very near future may not only have to bear their young without the aid of ancient folk rituals, but also without the support of modern maternity units and medicine.

The belly dance is believed to be the oldest form of childbirth preparation in the world, as the movements of the dance provide excellent exercise during pregnancy and aid natural childbirth during the final stages of labour.

In the Middle East, children who are taught the dance movements from a very early age have greater control of their abdominal muscles and pelvic area than Western women. Having mastered all the dance movements with dexterity, they are subsequently able to approach childbirth physically and mentally prepared.

Many problems that arise during pregnancy and labour can be directly caused by fear of childbirth and lack of correct preparation. Therefore it is extremely important to prepare physically and mentally for the great event.

Muscles should be toned up and strengthened by gradual and gentle exercise, preparing them for the work they have to do and to help minimise pain during labour. When the muscles have been toned up and strengthened, the effort of the womb will not be hindered, and as a result labour will be less painful and difficult. Correct exercise during pregnancy also enables the mother-to-be to take an active, helpful role in labour, and give birth without the need for drugs. There is also a great deal of self-satisfaction in being conscious as the baby is born.

In preparation for labour and the postnatal period, certain

movements of the belly dance can help tone up the muscles that support internal organs and strengthen the abdominal wall, which is continually being stretched during pregnancy to accommodate the growing baby. These movements will also encourage the opening of the pelvis, and the complete range of movement of the pelvis, as well as aiding the location of specific muscle groups and stretching and strengthening the pelvic floor.

Pelvic girdle pain or SPD pelvic pain (symphysis pubis dysfunction) is when the two halves of the pelvis which are connected to the front by a stiff joint called the symphysis pubis and a network of very strong ligaments, which under normal conditions allow very little movement to occur, loosen.

Normally these joints are not designed to allow movement, but when a woman becomes pregnant a hormone called relaxin is produced, which loosens the ligaments of the pelvis in order to allow slight movement of the pelvis at the time of birth. If these ligaments loosen too much and too early before birth, the stability of the pelvic joints becomes impaired, which leads to pain and inflammation in the pubic area and the groin.

Pain is also experienced in the inner thighs, buttocks and sacroiliac joints and hips when walking, turning over in bed, getting in and out of a vehicle, or climbing the stairs.

Kathy, one of my learners, described that feeling: it was as though her pelvis was coming apart. She felt unable to pick her feet up more than an inch off the floor, and from about 13 weeks couldn't sit down. The weight of her body also put pressure on her pelvis which was very painful. For 6 months she was advised to wear a belt around her pelvis, tie her legs tightly together, and not to climb stairs. Despite this debilitating problem throughout two pregnancies, happily she gave birth to two beautiful healthy daughters.

Physiotherapists are very supportive of the belly dance movements, because they tone and strengthen the core muscles of the abdomen on which all female organs sit. Specific movements for SPD include stomach exercises such as tummy rolls and flutters, camel rocks, back bends and circles. It's very interesting to find that many belly dance movements are possible. Some women with SPD find that circling their hips is comfortable even when they have been told to restrict their movements, despite their problems.

The lumbar region of the spine can become painful due to the continually increasing weight one is carrying around the middle when pregnant. But doing regular low-impact belly dance movements during pregnancy will help strengthen the core muscles around your stomach and help relieve pain and discomfort in the lumbar region.

Weak abdominal muscles cause backache, as they have to support the spine while the body is upright. A slack and weak pelvic floor can cause a collapse of the womb, which is known as a prolapse of the uterus. If the tone of the muscles is weak or is strained during pregnancy or birth, they are unable to support the uterus, which slips down into the vagina. However, this condition will respond to medical treatment.

During birth, the outlet of the birth passage dilates or opens to such an extent that the muscles of the pelvic floor become greatly overstretched, and as a result some women require stitches.

The pelvic floor muscles which surround and support the vagina, urethra and anus are designed to aid micturition (urinating), defecating (opening the bowels) and childbirth. If these pelvic floor muscles are lax when pregnant, you may find difficulty in controlling your bladder and experience other problems.

Pelvic floor exercises will not prevent lacerations, but they will help to stretch and strengthen the pelvic floor during pregnancy and the postnatal period, by helping to tone up and relax the pelvic floor. Muscles should only be stretched gently during uterine contractions and relaxation. The uterine muscles are controlled by hormones and cannot be controlled by working them yourself.

The recti muscles which run from top to bottom of the abdomen often divide during pregnancy, therefore practising gentle movements of the belly dance postnatal will help bring them back together. If the muscles are toned up and strengthened by doing gentle belly dance movements, the effort of the womb will not be hindered, and labour will be less difficult and painful and therefore the birth process will be eased.

Fighting against contractions will only produce more pain during labour. During pregnancy the abdominal walls and skin stretch considerably to accommodate the baby. If your muscle tone is weak, the muscles will not contract back to their normal shape after the birth and you will end up with a flabby tummy. Provided you have a trouble-free pregnancy, abdominal rolls and tummy flutters can be practised after the first 12–16 weeks. These movements are not only soothing for the baby but will help to tone up the abdominal muscles.

The dynamic, natural and instinctive rhythmic movements of the belly dance particularly benefit pregnant women, and getting in touch with one's own unique rhythm is an excellent preparation for labour. Even the sexy nature of some of the movements helps release hormones which are beneficial. This is particularly true in labour, probably because the production of oxytocin is encouraged.

Belly dance movements, when combined with breathing, yoga techniques and visualisation, help to release natural endorphins and induce a 'trance'-like state which optimises stamina, and acts as pain relief.

These movements also help release stress and gently promote stamina in mid-pregnancy, which is good for the mother-to-be in helping to build up physical strength. Combined belly dance and arm movements strengthen the middle and upper back, support heavier breasts, and make space for the diaphragm and baby, as baby grows. Gentle belly dance movements will also help to keep the weight down. Annoyingly, excess weight can cause ugly stretch marks, although a tendency to stretch marks is also determined by skin type.

Emotionally, gentle belly dance movements not only open up the heart and are enjoyable, but can be done with one's birth partner and used in labour, for example hip rotations/circles, the most basic of belly dancing movements, figure eights and hip sways, pelvic rocks and camel rocks. Even hip shimmies can be practised during the very final stages of labour. Working with gravity helps the baby to engage in the pelvis in late pregnancy and supports contractions, for example opening the cervix while in labour.

If you can maintain a sensible fitness programme of gentle belly dance movements throughout pregnancy, you should return to normal very quickly after the birth.

After the birth the vaginal and anal muscles become slack, which could affect your sex life. However, if you practised the movements of the belly dance and antenatal exercises that help tone up the pelvic floor and vaginal muscles, this problem should not arise. If the latter does not apply to you, the dance movements will generally tone up those muscles, enabling you to contract and relax at will, which will ultimately improve and enhance your sex life for you and your partner.

In some parts of the Middle East when a mother-to-be is about to give birth, she adopts a position that is sometimes performed by belly dancers when doing the floor dance. From a kneeling position the woman lowers her bottom to the floor, places her feet on either side of her thighs, then leans back very gently until her head and shoulders rest on the floor. Once in this position her body begins to relax. She is then encouraged to breathe slowly and rhythmically followed by fast shallow breathing, which increases with each contraction and produces abdominal movements such as belly rolls and ripples. The upper part of the roll is done between contractions of the womb, and the lower roll is done as the womb contracts, aiding the baby's entrance into the world with minimum stress on muscles and internal organs. Many mothers-to-be who have adopted this position found it surprisingly relaxing. But please, do not try this position unless aided by a childbirth expert.

Numerous women around the world now prefer a natural birth without the aid of drugs, enjoying the satisfaction of being conscious when the baby is born. Many of my students who have belly danced their way through pregnancy and labour have been back in class with their baby within 2 or 3 weeks, feeling absolutely wonderful and looking great.

Advice: If you have exercised regularly, i.e. done yoga, belly dancing or any other form of dance or exercise before becoming pregnant, you can continue what you are doing at the same level when you become pregnant. If you have not done any form of exercise or dance up until your pregnancy, you must be 12 weeks pregnant before commencing any form of dance or attending a course in belly dancing. Please seek advice from your doctor, antenatal teacher or a women's health clinic.

The National Childbirth Trust is a registered charity (801395) and if you have any concerns relating to your pregnancy or birth experiences you can contact any of the following NCT helplines for information or to speak to a qualified antenatal teacher or counsellor.

Pregnancy and Birth Line: 0300 330 0772, 9am – 8pm, Monday to Friday

Breastfeeding Line: 0300 330 0771, 8am – 10pm, seven days a week

Postnatal Line: 0330 330 0773, 9am – 1pm, Monday to Friday

Shared Experience Line: 0330 330 0774, 9am – 3pm, Tuesday, Wednesday and Thursday

(Sources: Barbara Watterson, *Women in Egypt*, Alan Sutton

Publishing; Monica Sjoo and Barbara Mor, *The Great Cosmic Mother*)

20. Hysterectomy

In the UK approximately 60,000 women ranging in age between their thirties and sixties will, in any given year, have a hysterectomy. The only organ removed during a hysterectomy is the womb which is a major muscle group but is not a stomach muscle nor a part of a stomach muscle. The only other organs that can be removed are the ovaries and fallopian tubes.

The top of the vagina may sometimes be removed and, if cancer has been diagnosed, the broad ligaments are removed. However, when an *abdominal* hysterectomy is performed, damage occurs to the abdominal muscles because the incision has been performed through the outer layer of the abdomen which is not the case with *vaginal* or *laparoscopic* hysterectomies.

If both your ovaries and uterus are removed, you may experience menopausal problems, for which your doctor may recommend oestrogen replacement therapy. You may also experience some emotional issues, including depression, or find that your desire for sex has diminished since your operation.

The women I have spoken to told me that having a hysterectomy was the best thing they ever did as it has improved the quality of their lives and they still enjoy an active and satisfying sex life.

Your gynaecologist/consultant will advise you against doing any form of exercise for at least 3 months in order to give you time to fully heal. But when you get the all-clear then you can join a belly dance class for a good core workout. You will find the movements that concentrate on the lower half of your body very beneficial to your health and general well-being as they will increase the production of endorphins, lessen tension and depression, tone up those abdominal muscles which support and surround internal organs, stretch and strengthen the pelvic floor which will help maintain the functions of the body, and also help to improve your sexual energy.

A few years ago I met a great character, a very famous singing gynaecologist, when we both appeared on a couple of TV programmes together. He said to me that if every female from a young age did belly dancing there wouldn't be so many flabby tummies, nor so many gynaecological problems.

For help, support and advice contact The Hysterectomy Association, or consult your doctor.

Email: info@hysterectomy-association.org.uk (telephone line discontinued due to costs)

21. Awareness of breathing

Appreciate the life-giving air
We must be aware
Someday each of us will take our last breath.
The cool air rushing inwards
Reminds us to appreciate
Our breath
Our Life.
(Ed McGaa Eagle Man, *Mother Earth Spirituality*)

Few people know how to breathe correctly or are aware that a lack of oxygen due to poor breathing techniques leads to numerous dysfunctions such as poor circulation which affects our vital organs and cells, plus other health problems such as anxiety, stress, tension in the neck and shoulder muscles, headaches, migraine, lethargy, poor concentration, loss of memory and a weak immune system.

For those of you who suffer from asthma, controlled diaphragm breathing is vitally important in helping to manage and improve your condition because it helps to strengthen the lungs and chest muscles which become weak because they are overworked; it also aids the reduction of mucus congestion.

Since I began teaching belly dancing, I have introduced the Buteyko method of correct breathing techniques; it has helped to improve many learners' asthmatic condition.

Changing the pattern of how we breathe leads to good health and well-being. When we breathe correctly our bodies get the full amount of oxygen they require and it also helps the removal of carbon dioxide which improves our immune system, general well-being and lifestyle. It is not necessary to inhale or exhale deeply; the slower and gentler you breathe, the more oxygen you inhale and the calmer and less stressed you become.

Most of us tend to breathe with short, shallow breaths from the top portion of our chests, which stresses our bodies, particularly the shoulders and neck that become overused and inflexible. The top of the lungs is narrow and small, therefore the amount of oxygen exchange is minimal. If you breathe correctly it allows you to fill your lungs with air from top to bottom. It is important to use the diaphragm, a dome-shaped muscular partition between the chest and the abdomen, which is attached to the ribs.

When you breathe in, the thorax expands, causing the diaphragm to descend and flatten out. This increases the capacity of the lungs; therefore we get the maximum amount of air into our lungs. This is sometimes called 'belly breathing' because, as the diaphragm comes down, it pushes the abdomen out (the abdomen is situated between the diaphragm and pelvis). When you breathe out, the thorax contracts and the diaphragm is raised, pushing the stale air out of the lungs. Gentle and regular breathing rapidly increases your oxygen supply, and stimulates the circulation, helping to keep the muscles healthy. It also helps you to raise your energies, relax, release stress and reduce tension in the shoulders and neck. Breathing correctly also improves your complexion and enhances your looks.

Tummy exercises using the diaphragm are often used in the belly dance, sometimes in a slow controlled way with abdominal rolls. Rhythmically pushing your stomach in and out or doing a quick flutter helps to firm up the tummy muscles and prevent flabby tummies.

When doing breathing exercises, always keep your back straight and don't wear anything too tight around your waist or tummy, as this will restrict your abdominal breathing. Physiotherapists also treat some back pain patients with abdominal breathing exercises which are known as 'diaphragmatic breathing'.

If you feel light-headed when doing any of the following breathing exercises, relax for a few minutes, then continue. This happens because you're increasing the oxygen levels to your brain.

It is important to do some gentle warm-ups such as the arm movements or hip circles on pages 73 and 133 before commencing with your breathing exercises. The majority of learners attending dance or fitness classes and some teachers are not aware that some breathing exercises are quite strenuous as you use many muscles.

The intercostals are muscles composed of several groups of muscles which run between the ribs and assist in forming and moving the chest wall, for example, helping to expand and contract the chest cavity as you breathe in and out.

You can do the following exercise standing; or, lying comfortably on your back, draw up your knees till slightly bent, keeping your feet flat on the floor and arms down by your side.

But do make sure your back is aligned correctly before beginning, i.e. your head is in line with your feet. If you are lying down, you may feel yourself drifting off, which is great as you are relaxed.

Breathing techniques

Experts now believe that breathing through an open mouth is not correct and you should only breathe in and out through your nose; with practice you will soon get used to this method of breathing. Many years ago, even though I found it difficult and a little uncomfortable at first, I found this method of breathing helped to relieve my blocked nose, and that's before I heard about the Buteyko method of breathing whose details I have included.

To prepare yourself for the following breathing exercises you should be relaxed and calm. Close your mouth lightly and continue to do so throughout the breathing exercises unless instructed otherwise.

Breathing exercise 1: Nasal breathing

a) As you slowly, gently and smoothly inhale through your nose, push your tummy out.

b) As you slowly and smoothly exhale through your nose pull your tummy in.

Repeat several times.

Exercise 1a

Or as you breathe in pull your tummy in and as you breathe out push your tummy out.

Breathing exercise 2

You will need to stand for this one.

a) As you slowly and gently inhale through your nose, push your tummy out and down.

b) Hold for a count of four.

c) As you slowly and gently exhale through your nose, lift your tummy up and pull in.

Repeat several times.

Breathing exercise 3

Stand for this breathing exercise which is the basic exercise for helping you to roll your belly.

a) As you inhale gently through your nose, pull your tummy in, then up; hold for a count of four.

b) As you begin to exhale through your nose, push your tummy out, then down.

Repeat several times from (a) to (b).

Breathing exercise 4

When doing this in class there are always fits of giggles among the learners as they observe one another's facial expressions.

Make sure your spine is aligned by raising your rib cage and holding your head up.

a) Close your mouth and place your thumb on the right side of your nose to block your right nostril.

b) As you inhale through your nose, push your tummy out.

c) Placing your index finger very lightly on your left nostril, exhale through your nose as you pull your tummy in.

d) Block your right nostril again with your index finger and repeat several times from (a) to (c).

Repeat several times.

Exercise 4a

Or as you breathe in pull your tummy in and as you breathe out push your tummy out.

Breathing exercise 5

Stand and keep your spine aligned by raising your rib cage and holding your head up. This is also a good exercise for singers and swimmers.

a) Gently and smoothly inhale through your nose and hold your breath.

b) Now, very slowly, exhale through your nose and as you do, count in seconds until you have completely exhaled. How many counts did you manage? 24–30 plus? If so, well done. 16–20 – not so good; 10 or less – oh dear, you definitely need to improve. But don't despair; with practice you will be able to reach 30 and even 40 plus!

Breathing exercise 6: The diaphragm flutter
This is a great breathing exercise for asthmatics.

If you place the palm of your hand lightly on your diaphragm (the space between your stomach and rib cage) you will be able to feel your stomach moving in and out while you practise. The secret is to hold in your breath as you flutter your diaphragm.

a) Inhale through your nose and open your mouth slightly and, while holding your breath, pant very lightly and quickly through your mouth for as long as you can before running out of breath. If you are doing this correctly your diaphragm will flutter.

Relax, then repeat the exercise until you are able to flutter your stomach quickly and continuously without too much effort and smile at the same time!

Breathing exercise 7: Tummy
a) Assume starting position.
b) Close mouth gently.
c) Inhale through your nose.
d) Hold your breath, then...
e) Push your tummy out, then immediately pull your tummy in, repeat as many times as you can, then breathe out through your nose as you push your tummy out, and relax.

Asthmatics: a new way of breathing
It's believed some asthmatics could benefit from simple breathing techniques. The Russian professor Konstantin Buteyko

devised a series of special breathing exercises to normalise breathing, therefore normalising the level of carbon dioxide, and developing a new breathing method. Linda Meads, an improved asthma sufferer and a practitioner member of the Buteyko Institute of Breathing, believes that some asthmatics can greatly reduce symptoms and restore normal breathing patterns, by practising this series of specially devised simple breathing techniques to bring over breathing within the normal range, along with education on medication, foods, sleep and gentle exercise. She believes that bad breathing patterns are very common, and views them as the root cause of asthma, although this is believed by some to be a very controversial thought.

By practising the breathing techniques regularly, sufferers will greatly reduce symptoms, restore normal breathing patterns, and reduce reliance on medication. Numerous asthmatics have benefited greatly from attending belly dance classes combined with these simple breathing techniques. So if you are looking for ways of reducing symptoms and medication, you could also benefit from breathing retraining courses.

How can I tell if I breathe too much?

Professor Buteyko developed the following test to measure your depth of breathing and consequent levels of blood carbon dioxide. This method is called the Control Pause.

1) Sitting down close your mouth and breathe normally through your nose for a couple of minutes.
2) Take a normal breath in through your nose.
3) Allow a normal breath out through your nose.
4) Gently close your nose with thumb and forefinger and start to count the seconds.
5) When you feel the first need to breathe, release the nose and take a breath in through your nose. Keep the mouth closed at this point.
6) The number of seconds that have passed is your Control

Pause.

7) If you managed less than 10 seconds you have health problems.

8) If you can hold for less than 25 seconds your health needs attention.

30–40 seconds is satisfactory. 40–50+ seconds is excellent.

If you are interested in the Buteyko method of breathing, contact them by telephone on this UK number: 0800 376 8361. You can also order the book, *Close Your Mouth: The Buteyko Breathing Clinic Self-Help Manual – Stop Asthma, Hay Fever and Nasal Congestion Permanently*, by Patrick McKeown.

22. Muscle tone

Lack of activity destroys the good condition of every human being, while movement and methodical physical exercise save it and preserve it.
(Plato)

Tense muscles affect our posture, and can be related to other discomforts such as back pain and neck ache, gynaecological problems, headaches, insomnia, fatigue, irritability, premature ageing, sluggish circulation, plus much more, which as a result can change our whole outlook and quality of life in our everyday activities, such as relationships, emotions and mental stability.

Intense slow movement helps to improve muscle tone, particularly those that surround and support the internal organs and pelvic floor. During exercise, muscles contract, and the more we make demands upon our muscles, the stronger they become.

Stress can cause a shortening of some muscles, which could shorten our whole structure. It is very important for your health and general well-being to maintain and improve muscle tone and strength in order to improve your posture balance, loosen those stiff joints and relieve the stress.

The muscles' function is to move the joints, which are attached to the end of the bones by ligaments; according to the origin and insertion near a joint, they perform a specific movement. The ends of the bones are protected by cartilage, and a capsule of synovial membrane surrounds them.

Muscles work in groups and when they become idle they become weak, and lose their elasticity and strength. They also become flabby and have to be retrained to function effectively. If you discipline your muscles steadily to their full capacity, your flexibility will improve greatly. You will also find that good muscle tone will also loosen stiff joints and improve your balance.

What not to do is stand or sit with your legs crossed. My generation were told to keep our knees together and not to cross our legs, which can encourage thread veins. When we push our thighs together we damage muscles known as abductors, which causes them to become overstretched. To prevent this happening keep your knees slightly apart when sitting.

As mentioned in my previous book, *Belly Dance: The Dance of Mother Earth*, it is important to understand the difference between a tense group of muscles and a relaxed group of muscles, and be able to feel each group move independently from one another when learning to belly dance. Correct isolation should enable you to move one group of muscles without moving another. If isolations are done correctly, you should be able to move the upper part of your body without moving your lower half, and vice versa. Isolation must be mastered correctly; otherwise your posture and the dance movements will look uncontrolled and ungainly. Assuming the starting position as instructed before commencing with any exercises and dance movements is important.

Belly dancing must be the best workout ever for your 'abs' and core strength ability, stabilising the spine and pelvis, helping to create balance and symmetry of movement. The core consists of your abdominal muscles (the transverse abdominus, rectus abdomini) and also includes the obliques, lower back and glutes, representing the area of your body that co-ordinates movement.

Fats, carbohydrates and protein are very important for your body and enable your body to function properly. If you cut any of these out, your body will break down. Your body needs a certain amount of fats to enable it to function properly, so do not cut out all fats. Seek advice about this.

The muscles that surround and support your internal organs also need exercising. Pelvic floor exercises such as pelvic tilts, hip circles, figure eights, stomach rolls and flutters are some of the best movements you can do to stretch and strengthen the muscles of the pelvic floor and maintain a healthy gut. Strong pelvic floor muscles have a positive effect on your large intestine as they contract and relax the colon which helps to eliminate the waste from your gut effectively, and controlled diaphragm breathing will also help.

The movements of the belly dance which concentrate on the lower parts of the body (the pelvic region) release the energy block of the solar plexus situated between the twelfth thoracic vertebra and the first lumbar vertebra.

For thousands of years tribal communities used the concept of dance to induce some kind of relief from emotional stress, anxieties, certain ailments and diseases of the stomach, which were believed by them to be an invasion of demons. These they exorcised through frenzied, contorted and convulsive forms of dance until they collapsed from sheer exhaustion.

The ancient shamans discovered that reactivating this area known as the navel chakra, which is also called the solar plexus or *hara*, had a positive effect on diseases of the stomach as well as creating a feeling of well-being.

Activation of the sacral chakra, situated between the fifth lumbar vertebra and sacrum, helps to improve pre-menstrual tension, and menstrual and menopausal problems, by harmonising the body's fluids, which has a positive effect on the urinary tract and blood diseases, and can also help to ease arthritis. By concentrating on the base chakra between the sacrum and coccyx, tension is reduced in the spine, and the nervous central system is calmed down.

(Sources: Holger Kalweit, *Dreamtime and Inner Space*, 1984; Tina Hobin, *Belly Dance: The Dance of Mother Earth*, 2003)

23. Posture

The spine is the tree of life; respect it.
(Martha Graham speech, 1965)

Correct posture is extremely important in helping to improve and maintain a healthy life. Incorrect posture can be seen in people with bulging bellies, round shoulders and head carried too far forward, a dropped rib cage, limping, or walking flat-footed. Dancing regularly in high-heeled shoes can also be related to back pain. Incorrect posture puts a strain on other parts, giving rise to further muscle strain which will cause backache and discomfort in other joints, due to the imbalance of the body's posture. Poor posture can also relate to how you project yourself and give an insight into your personality.

There are various types of bad posture, but the main ones are:

- Straight back with insufficient curve
- Loss of lordosis, which is the hollow in the lower back
- Scoliosis – a sideways curve of the spine
- Kyphosis – a rounding of the upper part of the back
- Poke neck – posterior pulling of the spine in the neck

Some students tend to complain of an aching hip when dancing; this can be due to leaning and putting weight on one side which causes a twist of the spine. To alleviate this problem always make sure your weight is evenly distributed on both feet when standing and your posture is correct when dancing or exercising. However, if the pain persists, make an appointment to see your doctor as it could be due to the early onset of arthritis or other problems.

Rolling the feet inwards is a very common problem among students and one that is seldom corrected. Rolling the feet inwards causes the bone in the lower leg (the tibia) to pivot inwards, which forces your pelvis to tilt forward, and increases the hollow in your back, which can result in low back pain. Rolling the feet outward and inward excessively can also cause knee pain. So, always make sure your weight is evenly distributed by holding the feet firmly to the floor when standing or dancing on the spot and travelling forward or when walking.

The feet have five metatarsal bones, which spread out across the foot in front of the mid foot. The shape of the bones in the feet fit together to make an arch which the heel bones sit behind, and when you're standing, take some of the body weight. The rest of your weight is supported by the first metatarsal, which is connected to the big toe, and fifth metatarsal, which is connected to the little toe.

These three arches of the foot are connected to three major weight-bearing points and when held to the floor disperse your weight evenly.

Many belly dancers wear high-heeled shoes when performing, but this is not recommended as it will eventually lead to back problems.

The gentle curve in your lower back is a natural hollow known as lordosis. If your posture is bad it can cause your back to curve inwards more than it should do naturally. This is described as an exaggerated lordosis, a contraction of the lumbar vertebrae.

Never stand, do exercises, or dance with your knees locked. Not only does adopting this stance restrict freedom of movement, making belly dance movements very difficult to do, but it can also encourage your lower spine to curve inwards more than it should. Just as an experiment, lock your knees and place your hand on the lower part of your back just below your waistline. Can you feel the exaggerated hollow? Keep your hand in the same position, elevate your rib cage and flex your knees – feel the difference? You should now be able to feel a much gentler natural curve in your lower back.

Lordosis posture can be helped by doing several pelvic tilts on a daily basis, a movement which will help to strengthen the abdominal muscles and correct spinal lordosis.

When belly dancing, many learners have a tendency to lean back which is a bad habit and should immediately be discouraged by teachers. When you lean back you are extending and compressing the joints, which could lead to lower back problems. To prevent muscle strain and low back problems always be aware of your posture and adopt the starting position: rib cage elevated, shoulders down, knees slightly relaxed and both feet firmly on the floor.

Many learners when beginning classes experience low back pain, the explanation being that the sacrum, which is part of the backbone, has not been used to its full potential. So when doing the belly dance movements for the first time, the sacral vertebra begins to move correctly; this may cause a little strain and low back pain for a short time. However, if this pain persists for 2 or 3 weeks see your doctor, who may recommend a physiotherapist.

Chris, one of my senior learners, has had ankylosing spondylitis since her twenties. Her posture is very poor and therefore she finds difficulty in standing with her back aligned and her head up. When I met her at a party, I suggested belly dancing would help her, so she agreed to give it a couple of weeks but actually attended classes for several months. The transformation in her posture improved dramatically as did her flexibility. Even the other learners noticed the difference and made positive and encouraging remarks.

Slow Exercise

Those who do not find time for exercise will have to find time
for illness.

(Earl of Derby)

The following slow low-impact exercises are a good cardiovascular workout which can help to build up your cardiovascular
strength, enable you to make full use of your muscles in a proper
co-ordinated way, tone up muscles which surround and support
internal organs, stretch and strengthen the pelvic floor, and
improve joint mobility. They will also strengthen your upper
body, help to release the blocked energy of the solar plexus,
improve your circulation, balance, co-ordination and stamina,
and prepare you overall for belly dancing.

Try to plan a regular time for your workout which should
only be done on alternate days. Decide which exercises you are
going to concentrate on, then do the warm-ups. Choose an airy
room with as much space as possible, make sure there is nothing
you can bump into, and remove any rugs to avoid tripping or
slipping on them. If the weather is favourable you could do your
exercises outdoors.

It is not necessary to play music when exercising as you may
be tempted to try and keep up with the rhythm. Neither should
you do any stretching exercises as a warm-up as they are very
strenuous and will strain your muscles, tendons and ligaments.
So, before you start any exercise or dance workout always do
some very gentle warm-up exercises first; just choose a few of the
following exercises as a warm-up. Arm movements are an ideal
warm-up as they help to stimulate and improve your circulation
and raise your oxygen levels.

To help your muscles work efficiently and allow them to
contract and release without stress, exercises should be done

smoothly, be controlled and not be too repetitive. When exercising, use your common sense and limit your sessions at first to allow your body to adjust without undue stress or strain. When you start using muscles that have hitherto been idle you must not overdo it. If you are generally out of condition or begin to feel tired and breathless, or experience aches and pains other than those you might ordinarily feel, you must stop and rest. Neither will you gain anything by over-exercising, or exercising too vigorously. Remember, aching and painful muscles are lacking in oxygen, so stop.

For many men and women exercise can become obsessional, a problem which is causing concern among health and fitness experts. Many believe that if you're not profusely sweating and your muscles aren't aching after exercising, you have not had a good workout. Over-exercising may lead to injury, eating disorders, depression and a breakdown of the immune system, which will make a person prone to colds, flu and other ailments. What causes dependency on physical activity has not yet been concluded. One theory put forward by researchers suggests that exercise addicts become dependent on endorphins, which are thought to relieve the dull pain of overworked muscles, an effect similar to pain-relieving drugs.

Note: Very few women realise the effects of low- or high-impact exercises, including dancing, exercising, jogging or running, without the support of a good bra or sports bra. Uncontrolled movement of the breasts strains fragile ligaments and tissue, and as a result the breasts eventually start to chaff, and sag, resulting in much pain and discomfort which may affect your posture. In some cases these problems can lead to long-term damage or to permanent damage of the breasts. So whether you have small or large breasts, protect them from injury by always wearing a good supporting bra when doing any form of dance or exercise.

Exercises

Starting position

Whenever you are asked to assume the 'starting position', you should, as instructed...

a) Stand with your feet close together, not touching, or as wide as your hip line.
b) Hold your feet firmly to the floor.
c) Flex your knees, i.e. bend them slightly.
d) Elevate your rib cage, i.e. lift your rib cage.
e) Hold up your head.
  If you have followed those instructions your spine should now be correctly aligned.

Exercises for Arms

Assume starting position for all arm exercises.

Exercise 1

a) Stand with feet apart no wider than your hip line.
b) Flex knees.
c) Elevate your rib cage.
d) Hold up your head.
e) Gently sway your arms forward up to shoulder level, then gently back.
f) Repeat several times, swaying your arms forwards and backwards.

Exercise 2

a) Place your arms down by your side.
b) Gently raise your arms forward and up until above your head, then bring them down and swing them back.
c) Gently sway your arms forward again until above your head, then bring them down and swing them back.
  Repeat several times.

Exercise 3

a) Gently lift your arms up out to the side and up until above your head.

b) Cross your arms while above your head.

c) While still crossed, bring them down to the tops of your thighs.

d) Swing out and up to the sides to shoulder level. Continue by raising your arms above your head, crossing your arms and bringing them down, then up to the sides at shoulder level.

Repeat several times.

Exercise 4

This is a great exercise for toning up those upper arms and can be done standing or sitting. Keep your arms straight; don't bend them at the elbow.

a) Hold your arms out to the sides at shoulder level.

b) Raise your arms up above your head until hands touch back to back.

c) Immediately lower your arms down to shoulder level with hands facing upwards.

d) Immediately raise and lower your arms again.

Do ten to fifteen, then relax. If you have done this exercise correctly you will feel those muscles in the upper arms tightening up.

Exercise 5: Arm circles

a) Hold your arms above your head.

b) Slowly bring both arms down to the right, then across your lower torso, up to the left and raise them until they are up above your head again.

Repeat this circular arm movement from right to left four or five times.

Now try it in the opposite direction:

a) Hold your arms above your head.

b) Slowly bring them down to the left, across your lower torso, up from the right, and raise them until they are up above your head again.

Repeat this circular arm movement from left to right four or five times.

Exercise 6: Arm sway

a) Raise your arms above your head.

b) Gently sway them just a little from side to side.

Repeat several times.

Exercise 7: Arm sway with bend

a) Raise your arms above your head.

b) As you sway your arms to the right, slightly bend from your waist to the right.

c) As you sway your arms to the left, slightly bend from your waist to the left.

d) As you continue to sway your arms alternatively to the right and left, bend a little further each time.

Exercise 8: Arm swing

a) Hold your arms out to the sides at shoulder level.

b) Swing your arms forward until the hands touch back to back.

c) Immediately swing your arms out to the side, then forward again as in (b).

Repeat several times.

Exercise 9: For upper arms

Assume starting position.

a) Stand with your feet apart no wider than your hip line.

b) Place your left arm down by your side.

c) Raise your right arm up above your head and slightly out to the side

d) Clench the fist of your right hand, then bend the arm from the elbow and slowly bring it down until it is behind your head.

e) Unclench your fist and raise your arm slowly until it is above your head and take it slightly out to the side again.

f) Repeat this exercise with your right arm from (a) to (e) several times. Then repeat the exercise with your left arm several times.

If you prefer to sit while doing this exercise, sit on a sturdy stool, and make sure you can place both feet flat on the floor.

Exercise 10: Self shoulder massage

This is a great exercise for massaging your shoulders and can be done sitting or standing.

a) Hold your arms out to the side at shoulder level and keep them straight.

b) Roll your arms inwards from the shoulders, then roll them back.

Repeat this as many times as you can, then relax.

Exercise 11: Shoulder drops

If you prefer to sit while doing this exercise, sit on a sturdy stool and make sure you can place both feet flat on the floor.

a) Raise your right shoulder, bring it forward and drop it.

b) Raise your left shoulder, bring it forward and drop it.

Repeat raising and dropping your shoulders alternatively, several times.

Exercise 12: The shrug

If you prefer to sit while doing this exercise, sit on a sturdy stool and make sure you can place both feet flat on the floor.

a) Raise both shoulders up as high as you can.
b) Hold for four counts.
c) Drop your shoulders and hold for four counts.
   Repeat six to eight times, then relax.

Neck Exercises

It's better to sit on a chair or on the floor to do the following exercises. But do make sure your back is aligned before you commence, by elevating your rib cage and placing both feet firmly on the floor, and continue to inhale and exhale gently through your nose.

Warning: If you have limited movement in the neck, never force the neck further than it will go when doing the following exercises; just move it as far as you can without feeling any stress or strain. Do not drop the neck back unless instructed by a physiotherapist. Never rush neck exercises, as they should always be done slowly and gently. At first you may feel some stiffness in the neck; however, if you begin to feel any pain or discomfort when doing any of the following neck exercises, then you should stop immediately. Remember, your neck supports the skull which is the heaviest bone in your body and is usually more prone to arthritis.

When you have finished your neck exercises, sit still for a few minutes to prevent dizziness.

Exercise 13: Neck turn

a) Turn your head slowly to the right.
b) Bring your head back slowly to central position.
c) Slowly turn your head to the left.
d) Bring your head back slowly to central position.
   Repeat six times, then relax.

Exercise 14: Neck stretch

a) Slowly lower your head until your chin almost touches

your chest.

b) Slowly raise your head.

Repeat six times, then relax.

Exercise 15: Neck stretch variation

If your movement is limited don't force your head down onto your shoulder; just lower it as far as you can without causing any discomfort.

a) Slowly and gently lower your head onto your right shoulder.

b) Slowly raise.

c) Slowly and gently lower your head onto your left shoulder.

d) Slowly raise.

Repeat six times.

Exercise 16: Head roll

a) Gently lower your head down, as near to your right shoulder as possible.

b) Gently roll your head over towards the left shoulder and raise.

c) From the left, gently lower your head down towards your left shoulder and roll it over towards the right shoulder and raise.

d) From the right, lower the head and roll it over to the left and raise.

e) Continue to gently roll your head from right to left, left to right, four times.

Relax.

Body Stretches

Exercise 17: Side stretches

a) Assume starting position.

b) Stand with feet close together but not touching.

c) Flex knees.

d) Elevate rib cage, drop shoulders down and hold your head up.

When doing the following stretch exercises, do not lean over to one side as you stretch. Keep your back straight throughout the exercise.

a) Raise your arms above your head and hold them in that position throughout the exercise.

b) Place your right foot forward, keeping the leg straight and heel raised.

c) Inhale gently through your nose as you slowly stretch your right side from toes to fingertips; hold for a count of four. (If you are doing this correctly, you will feel your rib cage pulling up and away from your pelvis.)

d) Exhale gently through the nose slowly as you relax to a count of four.

e) Place your right leg beside your left leg.

f) Place your left leg forward, keeping the leg straight and heel raised.

g) Inhale gently through the nose as you slowly stretch your left side from toes to fingertips. Hold for a count of four.

h) Exhale gently through your nose as you relax to a count of four.

i) Place your left foot beside your right foot.

Do at least three to four stretches on each side, then relax.

Exercise 18: Alternate side stretches

Follow the same breathing pattern as you did for the side stretches in exercise 17.

a) Assume starting position.

b) Feet close together but not touching. Keep your back straight; do not lean over to one side when stretching.

c) Raise your arms above your head and hold them in that position throughout the exercise.

d) Place your right leg forward, keeping the leg straight and heel raised.

e) Inhale slowly through your nose to a count of four as you slowly stretch your right leg and left arm at the same time.

f) Exhale slowly through your nose to a count of four as you relax and place your right foot beside your left foot.

Left side

a) Place your left leg forward, keeping the leg straight and heel raised.

b) Inhale slowly through your nose as you stretch your left leg and right arm at the same time.

c) Exhale through your nose as you relax to a count of four and place your left leg beside your right leg.

Do four stretches on each side.

Exercise 19: Limb and body stretch

This exercise should be done slowly and controlled while breathing in and out through your nose.

a) Assume starting position.

b) Stand with your legs apart at hip width and weight evenly distributed.

c) Hold both arms out in front of you and slowly bend forward, until your head is between your arms.

d) Stretch your body forward as far as possible without losing your balance and being careful not to dip your back. Your weight should be evenly distributed and your spine straight, not dipped. Do not bounce up and down as this can cause muscle tension in the thighs, and tear the hamstrings.

e) Hold to a count of six, then, very slowly, bring your arms down and stand upright. If you straighten up too quickly you may feel dizzy.

Exercise 20: Variation on limb and body stretch

a) Assume starting position.

b) Feet apart no wider than your hip line.

c) Both feet held firmly to the floor.

d) Bend forward, holding arms out in front of you with your head between your arms.

e) Stretch your body forward, being careful not to dip your back.

f) To complete a full circular movement with your right arm, bring your right arm down, and slowly push it up and out behind you.

g) Swing your right arm up and over till out in front of you again, back to the starting position.

h) Repeat with your left arm.

Continue the exercise using your arms alternatively. Do about ten to sixteen, then bring both your arms down and very slowly stand upright. If you come up too quickly you may feel dizzy.

Exercise 21: Body stretch

Assume starting position. Stand with your feet slightly apart, and held firmly to the floor.

a) Clasp your hands behind your back, resting them lightly on your buttocks.

b) As you slowly inhale through your nose, push your chest and chin out, stretching your arms back at the same time.

c) Hold for four counts. You should feel your rib cage pulling up and away from your pelvis.

d) As you slowly exhale through your nose, relax your arms, chest and chin.

Repeat four or five times.

Exercise 22: Seated spine stretch

If you find it difficult to place your hands flat on the floor, leave this exercise until you are more flexible; otherwise you may strain yourself.

a) Sit on a hard chair.

b) Hold both feet firmly to the floor.

c) Inhale through your nose as you slowly bend forward until you can place your hands on the floor alongside your feet.

d) Hold for about 7–10 seconds, or more if you can without stressing the spine, then as you exhale through your nose slowly come up until upright.

Repeat three or four times.

Exercise 23: Forward bend and stretch

Assume starting position. Feet apart, but no wider than your hip line, and weight evenly distributed.

Breathe as you did for exercise 22.

a) Raise your arms above your head.

b) Slowly bend forward until your fingertips reach your toes.

c) Come up slowly until into an upright position with arms raised and then bend forward again.

Repeat three or four times.

If you are flexible you should be able to touch your toes with your fingertips. If not, just bend forward as far as you can comfortably.

Exercise 24: Twist and bend

Assume starting position. Stand with feet apart as wide as your hip line and parallel.

This exercise must be done slowly, while inhaling and exhaling through your nose.

a) Hold your arms out to the side.

b) Twisting from your waist, bring your right arm across and down to your left foot.

c) Your left arm should now be up behind you.

d) Slowly, as you rise to an upright position, bring your right arm up and out to the side. You should be at starting position with both arms held out to the side.

e) Twisting from the waist, bring your left arm across and down to your right foot. Return to your starting position and repeat four or five times.

Exercise 25: Lateral bends

Assume starting position. Stand with your feet apart as wide as your hip line. Place arms down by your side.

Inhale slowly and gently through your nose as you bend. Exhale slowly and gently. Inhale through your nose as you straighten up.

a) Raise your right arm above your head.

b) Place your left arm down your left side with the right hand on your right thigh.

c) Slowly bend sideways to the left from the waist and, as you do, slide your left hand down your left leg.

d) Slowly straighten up and immediately bend over to the left again. Repeat four or five times.

e) Change arms so that your left one is raised above your head and your right one is down by your right side; now slowly do four or five bends sideways to the right.

Exercise 26: Upper body circle

This movement may make you feel a little dizzy when you swing the upper part of your body down, so lift your head; this should help prevent you from feeling dizzy. However, if you suffer from dizziness then do not do this movement. If you have a back problem or are not flexible in the back, do not arch back.

Assume starting position. Feet apart no wider than your hip line and held firmly to the floor.

Gently and slowly inhale through your nose as you bend either to the right or left, and gently and slowly exhale through your nose as you straighten up from either the right or left.

a) Slowly bend to the right, swinging the upper part of your body down and round your front over to the left.

b) As you slowly straighten up from the left, arch your back and continue the circular movement to the right.

Do three or four to the right, then repeat the movement in the opposite direction by bending to the left.

This movement is effectively done by some belly dancers when performing; they whip their upper body around in one large circle, followed by two smaller ones in quick succession and it looks very effective if you have long hair.

Lower Back Exercises

Note: If you have any back problems please seek medical advice before commencing any of the following back exercises.

The following two exercises help to open up the lower back and ease low back pain.

Exercise 27: For lower back

a) Sit on a hard-backed chair, well forward.
b) Place both feet firmly on the floor with feet slightly apart.
c) Inhale slowly and gently through your nose as you raise your rib cage.
d) As you exhale slowly and gently through your nose, simultaneously push down your rib cage and tilt your pelvis forward while keeping your bottom on the seat.
Inhale and repeat. Do this exercise five or six times, then relax.

Exercise 28: For lower back

a) Lie flat on the floor on your back.
b) Place your arms by your side.
c) Make sure that your head is aligned with your feet.
d) Draw up your knees and keep both feet flat on the floor.
e) Inhale through your nose.
f) As you exhale slowly through your nose, simultaneously push down your rib cage and tilt your pelvis up without

raising your bottom up from the floor.
Inhale and repeat several times.

Exercise 29: For abdomen and back

a) Lie flat on your back.
b) Legs straight and close together.
c) Place arms down by your side.
d) As you inhale slowly through your nose, press the middle of your back into the floor.
e) Exhale slowly through your nose and relax.
Repeat four or five times.

Exercise 30: Tip to toe stretch

Before commencing with the following three exercises, you must align your back, making sure that your head is in line with your feet.

a) Lie flat on your back.
b) Extend your arms behind your head, with legs together and out straight.
c) Inhale slowly through your nose as you slowly stretch the whole of your body from toes to fingertips; hold for a count of four.
d) To a count of four, exhale through your nose as you relax. Hold for a count of four before continuing the exercise. Repeat the exercise four or five times.

Exercise 31: Side stretches

a) Lie flat on your back.
b) Extend your arms behind your head, with legs together and out straight.
c) Before you start your stretches, make sure that your head and feet are aligned.
d) Slowly inhale through your nose as you stretch your right side from your toes to your fingertips.

e) Hold to the count of four, then exhale through your nose as you slowly relax.

f) Do four or five of these stretches on the right side.

g) Repeat the exercise on your left side four or five times.

Exercise 32: Alternate side stretch

a) Lie flat on your back.

b) Extend your arms behind your head, with legs together and straight. Before you start your stretches, make sure your head and feet are aligned.

c) Inhale through your nose as you slowly stretch your left leg and right arm at the same time.

d) Hold, count up to four, then exhale slowly through your nose as you relax.

e) Inhale as you slowly stretch your right leg and left arm at the same time.

f) Hold, count up to four, and then exhale slowly as you relax.

Do four or five stretches on each side.

For Pelvis and Buttocks

Pelvic exercises are excellent for stretching and strengthening the pelvic floor, toning the muscles of the pelvic floor, the buttocks and the knees. They are also excellent exercises to do when pregnant and for those with SPD. The gluteus muscle which forms your bottom is the largest muscle in your body and can become fatty, and as a result we get those awful flabby bottoms. The following exercise can be done standing, sitting or lying down.

When doing the following exercises, breathe gently in and out through your nose.

Exercise 33: For the buttocks

a) Tighten the cheeks of your bottom.

b) Relax the cheeks of your bottom.

c) Tighten and relax several times.

Once you have mastered the exercise, do it as quickly as you can. You can also do this exercise by lying flat on your back or on your side, either on the floor or on your bed. Draw your knees up, relax and contract and relax the muscles alternatively and as quickly as you can. Then practise contracting and relaxing the buttocks alternatively.

Exercise 34: Basic pelvic thrust

Assume starting position. Feet slightly apart, knees flexed and held in that position throughout the exercise. Do not move the knees to and fro. If you do, you will not be able to do the exercise correctly and will not gain any benefit from doing the exercise.

a) Stick out your bottom.

b) Push your pelvis forward.

c) Immediately push your pelvis back, then forward again.

Repeat several times until you can thrust your pelvis forward and backward smoothly and effortlessly.

Exercise 35: Buttock tone

This is another great exercise for toning up the bottom.

Assume the starting position as for the basic pelvic thrust in exercise 34.

a) Tighten your buttocks, thrust the pelvis forward and tilt upwards.

b) Relax the buttocks, then push back.

c) Tighten your buttocks, thrust the pelvis forward and tilt upwards.

d) Relax the buttocks, and then push pelvis back.

Repeat several times.

Exercise 36: Pelvic lift and buttock toner

Do not arch your back too high as you may strain your back.

Your weight should be supported by your shoulders.

a) Lie flat on your back, with your arms by your side, palms up, legs together. Make sure your head and feet are aligned before commencing this exercise.

b) Breathing in slowly through your nose, tighten your buttocks and lift your bottom off the floor, thrusting your pelvis up.

c) As you gently exhale through your nose, relax your buttocks as you slowly lower your bottom down onto the floor.

Repeat several times.

Exercise 37: Buttock toner

While breathing gently in and out through your nose...

a) Lie flat on the floor, arms out to the side.

b) Draw your knees up and keep your feet flat on the floor.

c) Without actually lifting your bottom off the floor, tighten your buttocks and tilt your hips up.

d) Relax your buttocks as you push them down onto the floor. Repeat several times, then relax.

Exercise 38: For the waist

Note: Inhale through the nose as you swing your legs over and exhale through your nose as you lift your knees.

a) Lie flat on your back.

b) Place your arms out to the side.

c) Draw up your knees, feet flat on the floor.

d) Keeping both legs together, slowly swing legs over to the right until your right knee touches the floor.

e) Slowly lift your knees and slowly swing both legs over to the left until the left knee touches the floor. Repeat several times.

Exercise 39: Rib cage lift

Note: Inhale through your nose as you push the rib cage forward and exhale through the nose as you lower your rib cage.

a) Lie flat on the floor with arms down by your side, legs together and straight. Make sure your head and legs are aligned.

b) Keeping your shoulders and buttocks on the floor, push your rib cage forward. If you are doing this correctly, your upper back will slightly arch up from the floor.

c) Relax, lowering the rib cage back to the floor. Repeat several times, then relax.

Note: The following two exercises are strenuous on the lower back, so if you suffer from low back pain do not attempt these exercises until your back feels stronger and more supple.

Exercise 40: The body lift

Each time you stretch your body, slowly inhale through your nose, and as you lower your body to the floor, slowly exhale through your nose.

a) Lie flat on your back, legs together and out straight.

b) Extend your arms behind your head and keep your head on the floor throughout the exercise.

c) Slowly arch your body up a little from the floor, supporting it only with your shoulders and heels, and gently stretch slowly.

d) Slowly lower your body to the floor and relax. Repeat four or five times.

Exercise 41: The bow

Warning: Do not do this exercise if you have a muscle strain, or a back, hip or neck problem.

As you slowly stretch, inhale through your nose, and as you draw up your knees exhale through your nose.

a) Lie on your right side with your arms extended behind your head.
b) Slowly stretch the whole of your body while arching your back, arms, head and legs so as to form a bow shape with your body.
c) Hold to a count of four.
d) Slowly draw up your knees, relax your arms and count up to four.
e) Do three or four stretches on your right side, then roll over and repeat on your left side, inhaling slowly as you stretch and exhaling slowly as you relax.

Exercise 42: Press-ups

Warning: Do not attempt this exercise if you have a back problem.

a) Lie on the floor on your tummy.
b) Place your hands on either side of your rib cage.
c) To raise your upper torso, push up until your arms have straightened (but not locked at the elbows), keeping your tummy and legs on the floor.
d) Hold for three counts, then slowly bend your elbows and lower your upper torso to the floor.
   Do three or four more, then relax.

When you have mastered this exercise, slowly inhale through your nose as you raise your upper torso and exhale slowly through your nose as you lower yourself to the floor.

Exercise 43: Feline press-ups

Warning: Do not do this exercise if you have low back or knee problems, unless advised by your physiotherapist, osteopath or chiropractor.

a) Kneel on the floor, bend forward and place your hands on the floor in front of you, keeping your arms straight but not locked.

b) As you inhale through your nose, contract your tummy muscles (i.e. pull your tummy in).

c) Push out your rib cage.

d) Exhale through your nose as you bend your arms, push your pelvis forward and lower your chest to the floor.

e) As you inhale through your nose, push up and slowly straighten your arms, pushing your bottom out and arching your back.

f) Hold for a count of four and repeat the exercise four times. When you repeat this exercise, slowly inhale as you bend your arms and lower your chest to the floor. Slowly exhale as you straighten your arms and relax.

For Legs and Knees

The following exercises not only tone up the leg muscles, but are good exercises for those with knee problems. If your knee problem is recent and you have been receiving treatment, do seek medical advice before commencing the following exercises. When doing the following exercises, gently inhale and exhale through your nose.

Exercise 44: For legs and knees

If you cannot lie on the floor, sit on a hard chair and place your legs on a solid pouffe or stool which is level with your chair. Or sit up on the floor with your legs straight out in front of you.

If you need to support your back, sit against a wall or a solid piece of furniture.

a) Extend your legs in front of you, close together

b) Pull your feet up towards you, immediately relax, and repeat ten times.

c) Relax for 1 minute, then do ten more.

If you are doing this exercise correctly, your heels should rise slightly up from the floor.

Exercise 45: For legs and knees

a) Lie flat on your tummy. Keep your legs together and out straight and make sure you are aligned. You can place your arms down by your side or on the floor above your head.

b) Curl your toes under and keep them in this position as you raise your legs up from the floor and stretch them to a count of four.

c) Keeping your toes curled, lower your legs to the floor. Repeat ten times, relax for 1 minute, then do another ten.

Exercise 46: For the legs

a) Lie on your back on the floor with legs together.

b) Raise your right leg up off the floor.

c) Bend the leg from the knee.

d) Straighten out the leg and lower to the floor.

e) Raise your left leg up off the floor and bend the leg from the knee.

f) Straighten the leg and lower to the floor. Do six to eight on each leg, then relax.

Exercise 47: For the calf muscles

You may wish to hold onto something solid to do this exercise. Assume starting position.

a) Feet close together and keep your weight evenly distributed.

b) Rise up onto the balls of your feet.

c) Keeping your heels raised and back straight, bend your knees slowly as far as you can, then...

d) Lower the heels to the floor and straighten the legs but do not lock your knees.

e) Rise up onto the balls of your feet and repeat the exercise. Repeat three or four times, then relax.

Exercise 48: For the calf muscles

You will need to have good balance for this exercise, so do not attempt to do it if your balance is poor.

a) Place a telephone directory on an even, flat floor surface.
b) Stand on the directory with your heels over the edge.
c) Raise your rib cage and drop your shoulders.
d) Keep your back straight or you will lose your balance.
e) Hold arms down by your side or out to the side.
f) Rise up onto the balls of your feet, then immediately lower your heels. Repeat several times.

If you are doing this correctly you really will feel those calf muscles stretching.

Exercise 49: For creaking knees

Ever crouched down for something and felt as though you would never get up again because of your knees? Then try this exercise; it can even be done in the bath. If you do the exercise regularly for a week or two, you should be able to straighten up without your knees creaking and groaning. However, if your joints are painful seek medical advice before practising this exercise.

a) Place your thumb and middle finger firmly on either side of your knee cap (the patella).
b) Bend and straighten out the leg.
   Repeat the exercise several times on the right leg, then do it on the left leg.

Exercise 50: Energy booster

This exercise always makes my students giggle. It is a great exercise for releasing all that blocked energy in the solar plexus, improving your circulation and rise in oxygen levels, thus raising energy levels. Choose a very lively piece of music to do this exercise to.

Assume starting position.

a) Feet apart as wide as your hip line, and weight evenly distributed.

b) Relax your knees.

c) Hold your arms out in front of you at waist level, palms facing upwards. Now here comes the tough bit...

d) Tighten your buttocks and hold them tight throughout the exercise. Do not relax them until you have completed the exercise.

e) Thrust your hips to and fro as in pelvic tilts in quick succession; the quicker you can do it, the better.

With practice you should be able to do at least 100 tilts a minute. Believe me, it can be done, so persevere.

When you have done as many as you can, look at your hands. If you have done it correctly they should look mottled, bluish or reddish in colour, and feel warm. Some learners experience a tingling sensation in their hands and/or fingers. Others feel this tingling sensation in their abdomen, legs and feet. These changes are caused by improved circulation and rise in oxygen levels.

For the Face and Neck

The following exercises are for toning up the facial muscles and firming the neck. They can be done sitting, standing or lying down.

Exercise 51: For facial and neck muscles

Practise lifting your bottom lip up and stretching it over your top lip, and then relaxing the lip. Repeat three or four times until you can get that bottom lip right up and over your top lip.

a) Now repeat the movement as quickly as you can, stretching your lower lip over your upper lip, then immediately relaxing the lip.

b) Repeat the movement in quick succession as often as you can, and then relax.

You should, if doing it correctly, feel those neck muscles

contracting and relaxing.

Exercise 52: For facial and neck muscles

a) Open your mouth as wide as you can.

b) Keeping it open, pull your mouth outwards as though you are trying to touch your ears with the corners of your mouth, relax, then immediately pull outwards again.

Do the exercise as quickly and as many times as you can. 100 a day is ideal for helping to keep that jaw line and neck from sagging!

For Vagina and Anus Muscles

For many women, belly dancing has greatly improved the intimate side of their life, both for themselves and their partner. But if you want to add a little extra spice to your life, try the following exercises which were given to me many years ago by well-known anthropologist Sheila Kitzinger, and friend Margaret Jones, an antenatal tutor. These exercises will help to tone up all those important muscles that have become slack due to childbirth, surgery or lack of exercise.

Exercise 53

a) Sit on a chair or on the floor.

b) Imagine you are holding a pencil between the cheeks of your bottom or vagina.

c) Now write your name. Hope it's not a long one!

Exercise 54

a) Tighten and relax your vagina without tightening the cheeks of your bottom.

b) Repeat several times!

Exercise 55

Now tighten the cheeks of your bottom without tightening the vaginal muscles.

Repeat several times.

Exercise 56: For the buttocks

Strengthening the muscles (the gluteal muscles) in your bottom is vitally important in helping to prevent knee and hip problems.

All too often I hear complaints from women about their bottoms being too big, too flabby or both, but I always tell them: the bigger the bum, the better for belly dancing! Anyway, here are some fun buttock-toning exercises to try that will definitely help tone it up and help to prevent problems.

a) Place a piece of paper or a coin (a large one!) between the cheeks of your bottom.

b) Now hold it there for as long as you can as you walk slowly around the room.

Exercise 57: Buttock exercise

a) Sit on the floor with your legs stretched out in front of you. You may balance a little better if you support your back against something.

b) Place your hands lightly on your knees.

c) As you squeeze the cheeks of your bottom, part your legs a little, then relax.

d) Repeat this exercise until your legs are wide apart.

e) Now repeat this exercise by squeezing your buttocks as you bring your legs a little closer together each time until back to the starting position. Repeat the whole exercise once more, then relax.

Exercise 58: Buttock exercise

This exercise can be done when lying on your back or side. If lying on your back, draw up your knees; place knees together gently. If lying on your side, draw your knees up slightly.

a) Slowly contract and relax your thighs alternatively.

b) Once you have mastered this move as in (a), move your thigh muscles as quickly as you can. It will feel like you are shimmying your thighs.

c) Now try adding a little thrusting movement of the pelvis at the same time.

Exercise 59: For buttocks and vagina

a) Lie flat on the floor.

b) Draw up your knees.

c) Place a pillow or cushion between your knees.

d) Now, as you press your knees together, tighten your buttocks and vagina.

e) Relax, and repeat several times.

Abdominal Exercises

The following tummy exercises will help prevent a flabby tummy by toning up the stomach muscles that surround and support internal organs and massage internal organs.

Warning: Don't do the following tummy exercises on a full stomach or after drinking a fizzy drink as you may end up with a stitch or even feel a little sick.

Exercise 60: Tummy pushes

You must keep your rib cage elevated for these exercises.

a) Assume starting position.

b) Flex knees; stand with feet slightly apart, and weight evenly distributed.

c) Place your hands lightly on your tummy.

d) As you inhale through your nose gently, push your tummy out as far as you can without straining it.

e) As you exhale through your nose gently, pull your tummy in; imagine you are trying to touch your spine with it.

f) Inhale through your nose and push your tummy out again. Repeat a few times, then relax.

Exercise 61: For flabby tummies

This is a good exercise for toning up those flabby tummy muscles.

Assume starting position. Stand with feet slightly apart and weight evenly distributed.

a) As you slowly inhale through your nose, pull your tummy in, in four stages as though going up four steps.

b) As you slowly exhale through your nose, push your tummy down in four stages as though you are going down four steps.

Repeat three or four times.

Exercise 62: Abdominal exercise

a) Stand with your feet slightly apart, weight evenly distributed and knees flexed.

b) Exhale gently through your nose as push your tummy out and down.

c) As you inhale gently through your nose, lift up your tummy and pull it in. If you have done this correctly, your stance will have changed, i.e. your knees will be bent a little more.

d) As you exhale gently through your nose, push your tummy out and down.

Repeat several times.

Exercise 63: Tummy rolls

a) Stand with your feet slightly apart with your weight evenly distributed, then elevate your rib cage.

b) As you slowly inhale through your nose, pull your tummy in. Imagine you are trying to touch your spine with it.

c) Still inhaling, pull your tummy up until under your rib cage, then...

d) As you slowly exhale through your nose, push your tummy out and down.

If you have done this correctly, you should have rolled your tummy in a circle. Continue to do this several times.

Exercise 64: Abdominal muscle exercise

This is a fun way to exercise those abdominal muscles and can even be turned into a party piece! It's also a good core workout.

a) Find a coin – a two-pence piece will do.
b) Roll up your top and lower the waistband of your skirt or trousers, so your abdomen is exposed.
c) Lie flat on the floor.
d) Place the coin just below your belly button.
e) Push your tummy in and out and see whether or not you can flip the coin.
f) If you don't succeed, place the coin a little further down below your belly button.

It has been known for dancers to balance a glass of wine on their bellies and, using abdominal muscle control, tip the wine from one glass into another glass. Honestly! Apparently such an act was televised on *The David Frost Show* in the UK many years ago.

Exercise 65: For the diaphragm

Assume starting position.

a) Place both hands lightly on your diaphragm which is just below your bust.
b) Inhale, hold your breath and pant very lightly and as quickly as you can through your mouth.
c) If you are doing this correctly your diaphragm should be gently fluttering.

Other exercises develop single powers and muscles.

The Belly Dance

Exercise is good for you, but, like everything else, it can be overdone.

(Anonymous)

Belly dance movements are based on the natural structure of the body, so there should be no stress or strain for those of you suffering from low back pain or ill health if you are doing the moves correctly and providing your practitioner has given his or her consent for you to begin a gentle exercise regime.

Combined with a correct breathing programme and improved posture, its wide range of graduated dance movements help to strengthen muscles, develop muscle control, encourage joint and tendon stabilisation, and mobilise stiff and aching joints. As a result there is an improvement in circulation and a rise in oxygen levels, which makes for healthy organs, and tones up the whole body, while the creative potential of the dance movements stimulates spiritual energy and relaxes the whole being.

Whether learning belly dance for health and relaxation, or with the aspiration of becoming a professional dancer, this ancient art harmonises our body, mind and soul, giving us an overall feeling of well-being that will enhance the quality of our lives.

Belly dance movements are probably the most effective core workout existing. Ever since I started teaching, both women and men have told me that since taking up belly dancing their low back pain had eased or completely disappeared. So what could be a better core workout than belly dancing to help keep your body stable and lessen the pain?

What is a core workout?
Core strength refers to the muscles that stabilise your spine and pelvis for the arms and legs to act on, which helps to create

balance and symmetry of movement. 'Abs', short for 'abdominal muscles', work the area from waist to hip, strengthening your stomach and back muscles, which in turn helps reduce low back pain.

The abdominal muscles are in two parts on either side of the belly button from the sternum to the pubis. They obliquely fit across like a corset on either side. The first one you use to sit up; the second one you use during twisting. Basically it means that by working your abs, you are keeping your inner body strong.

The core is a difficult one to explain and abbreviate but it basically means keeping your inner body strong which is done by having a good strong posture in your legs, hips, bum and back. If your body is strengthened in the correct way, you're more likely to have better posture, prevent injuries, and enjoy a better quality of life and general well-being.

Belly dance movements to do to improve your abs include:

- Hip rotations
- Figure eights
- Pelvic tilts
- Abdominal rolls and flutters
- Rib cage rolls, slides, circles and lifts
- Abdominal breathing exercises

If you do the exercises correctly as you breathe gently in and out through your nose, you will feel the abs being worked. Refer to page 61 for correct breathing techniques and page 71 for warm-up exercises.

Do not do any stretches before commencing this workout as you need to warm up gently to stimulate your circulation and increase your oxygen supply. If you don't, you will strain your muscles, tendons and ligaments. This applies to everyone, whether fit or unfit.

Relaxation

Learn to relax – your body is precious. Inner peace begins
with a relaxed body.
(Norman Vincent Peale)

Note: Before you begin your relaxation session, carefully read
through the instructions first and memorise them as best as you
can. There will be no benefits to be gained if you are constantly
referring to the instructions. It's easy to follow so it won't take
you long to get the gist of it. Switch off your mobile phone and
take the telephone off the hook. If it's one of those that make a
noise when off the hook then place a couple of cushions or
pillows over it to dull or block out the sound.

First Stage of Relaxation

Breathing pattern

Lie on the bed, or on the floor on a blanket or duvet if you wish,
put a pillow under your head, and get into a comfortable
position. Make sure your head is aligned with your feet, as this
will ensure your spine is straight. Place your arms down by your
side, uncross your legs, and close your eyes. If you possess a
mask then wear that or draw the curtains or pull down the blind.
If you cannot lie down, choose your most comfortable chair,
preferably a recliner, but do not slump, as you must keep your
spine straight.

Start by doing some diaphragmatic breathing and inhale
through your nose as you push your tummy out, exhale through
your nose as you pull your tummy in. Continue this process to
establish a slow, steady, relaxed, rhythmic breathing pattern,
allowing the abdomen to rise and fall freely. The slower you
breathe, the more oxygen you produce and the calmer you will

become. The calmer you become, the lower the blood pressure. As your muscles relax there will be less of a resistance to the flow of blood, reduced pressure on the brain, and an improvement in your circulation. Continue to breathe deeply and slowly until the whole of your body feels relaxed and heavy. If you haven't fallen into a deep sleep continue with the following relaxation routine, tensing and relaxing specific muscle groups as instructed, and continue breathing gently.

Relaxation Session

Concentrate on your right foot.

Tense your right foot for 6 seconds, then very gradually release the tension, letting the foot slowly sink into deep relaxation.

Concentrate on your left foot and do exactly the same with your left foot as you did with the right foot.

Now concentrate on both feet and, as you do, feel them getting heavier and heavier.

Concentrate on your right calf muscle.

Tense the calf muscle for 6 seconds, then very gradually release the tension, allowing the calf to slowly sink into deep relaxation.

Concentrate on your left calf and do exactly as you did with the right calf.

Now concentrate on both calves, feel them relaxing and getting heavier and heavier, as they sink into the floor or bed.

Concentrate on your right thigh muscle.

Tense your right thigh muscle for 6 seconds, and then very gradually release the tension, letting the thigh slowly sink into deep relaxation.

Concentrate on your left thigh muscle and do the same.

Now concentrate on both thighs and feel them relaxing and getting heavier.

Now concentrate entirely on both feet and both legs; feel them relaxing and getting heavier and heavier. Imagine you are trying to lift them, but you can't because they are much too heavy to lift.

Concentrate on your right and left buttocks at the same time. Tense them both for 6 seconds, then very gradually release the tension, letting the buttocks slowly sink into deep relaxation; feel them getting heavier and heavier, as they sink into the floor or bed.

Concentrate on your abdomen. Tense the muscles of your abdomen for 6 seconds, then very gradually release the tension, letting the muscles of the abdomen slowly relax; let it flop as much as it can flop, and feel it slowly relaxing.

Now concentrate on your buttocks and abdomen at the same time; feel them getting heavier and heavier as they completely relax.

Tense your back for 6 seconds, relax it, then feel it gravitating further onto the floor or bed.

Concentrate on your chest muscles. Tense your chest muscles for 6 seconds, then very gradually release the tension, letting the muscles of your chest slowly sink into deep relaxation.

Now concentrate on your shoulders. Tense both your shoulders for 6 seconds, then very gradually release the tension, allowing the shoulders to slowly sink into deep relaxation. Feel them getting heavier and heavier as they gravitate onto the floor or bed.

Concentrate on the upper and lower muscles of the right arm. Tense your right arm for 6 seconds, then very gradually release the tension, and feel the arm getting heavier and heavier as it slowly sinks into deep relaxation and feels very heavy.

Concentrate on your right hand. Clench your right hand for 6 seconds, then very gradually release the tension, allowing the hand to slowly sink into deep relaxation, and feel very heavy.

Now concentrate on your right arm and right hand; feel them getting heavier and heavier. Imagine trying to lift them up but they are so heavy you can't.

Concentrate on your left arm. Tense the arm for 6 seconds, then gradually release the tension, letting the arm slowly sink into deep relaxation and feel very heavy.

Concentrate on your left hand. Clench your fist for 6 seconds, then very gradually release the tension, letting the hand slowly sink into deep relaxation and feel very heavy.

Concentrate on your left arm and hand; feel them getting heavier and heavier.

Now concentrate on both arms and hands and imagine you are trying to lift them but you can't because they are so heavy.

Concentrate on the neck. Tense the muscles of your neck for 6 seconds, then very gradually release the tension.

Concentrate on your face. Tense all your facial muscles for 6 seconds, then very gradually release the tension, allowing your jaw to drop and your mouth to open slightly.

Concentrate on your eyes.
Tighten your eyes for 6 seconds, then very gradually release the tension. You may feel a little discomfort at the back of your eyes or around your eyes, but don't worry; it's your eye muscles trying to relax.

Now let your head relax; imagine it is sinking further and further into the pillow or into the back of your seat and feeling heavier and heavier.

Now concentrate on the whole of your body; feel it getting heavier and heavier as it gravitates onto the floor or bed.

While you continue to drift deeper and deeper into total relaxation, imagine you are in your very own special place. You could be on your own private beach, in a beautiful garden or woodland, or a favourite room. As you let your imagination run free, feel all your stress, tension, anxiety and fears draining away, flowing down through your body from your head and out of your toes.

Enjoy this tranquil, calm and relaxed state for as long as you can, then slowly, very slowly to avoid dizziness, open your eyes and orientate yourself; wiggle your fingers and toes. When you are ready to rise, roll over onto your right or left side, raise yourself up, then slowly sit upright. Remain in this position for a couple of minutes before standing up.

Self-Communing

I am light with meditation, religiose
And mystic with a day of solitude.
(Douglas Dunn, 'Reading Pascal in the Lowlands', 1985)

If you are worried about something, feel stressed or depressed, then it's time to practise some self-communing. It's so important to give yourself some time from your hectic schedule to collect your thoughts and calm down your inner turmoil.

Find yourself a quiet and secluded place away from others where you won't be disrupted and can totally relax. Wear clothes that are loose around the waist and items of clothing that feel comfortable. Remove your shoes, but if your feet feel cold put on a pair of socks; it's impossible to relax if your feet are cold. Switch off your mobile phone. Even better, leave it in another room.

Sit in your most comfortable chair, or lie down on your bed. Start by focusing on your breathing, breathing gently in through your nose and out through your nose, or if you prefer, through your mouth.

As you start to relax and your body begins to feel heavier, imagine you are in a peaceful, beautiful place where the sky is blue and the sun is shining, sitting on the sand, rocks or a beach chair in your very own private sandy cove, listening to the waves breaking onto the shore. Maybe you prefer to be in a garden surrounded by colourful, exotic, scented flowers, listening to the birds singing, or sitting beside a crystal-clear babbling brook. You may prefer to choose your own very special place, one that brings back fond memories.

Wherever you are, look up to the sky and imagine that a little white cloud is floating towards you. While it's hovering above your head, tell it your worries one by one, and watch that little white cloud getting darker and darker as it absorbs your problems. When you have finished, watch that little dark cloud float up and float far away, taking all your worries with it.

You can also do this by putting each worry in a chest. Unlock the chest, put in your worries, and when you have finished close the lid and lock the chest, then hide it away. Or imagine you have a small chest of drawers. Open one of the drawers, put a worry in, then close the drawer. When you have filled the drawers, hide the box away.

When you are ready, open your eyes; sit for a few moments to reflect. After completing any of the above sessions on relaxation or self-communing, you should now feel much fitter mentally and physically, and able to face up to just about anything that's thrown at you!

Part II

Belly Dancing for Teachers and Learners

Safe and Effective Dance Practice

It is the supreme art of the teacher to awaken joy in creative expression and knowledge.
(Einstein)

There are many guidelines and techniques teachers should be proficient in before even thinking about starting to set up classes, as there is much more to teaching than just standing in front of a group and demonstrating a few belly dance movements to music. Unfortunately too many teachers lack teaching skills and safe and effective dance practice, which can put you, as a learner, at risk. The following information will give you as a learner an insight into what you should expect of your teacher.

Teachers should:

- Be aware of health and safety issues and the implementation of guidelines
- Be able to perform and demonstrate Middle Eastern dance to an appropriate standard of competence
- Advise you the learner on the physiological and spiritual benefits of the dance
- Demonstrate competence in teaching techniques, course design and delivery of the dance
- Have the ability to plan and deliver teaching programmes and learning sessions
- Perform and demonstrate all styles of the dance to a high standard of competence
- Impart knowledge with confidence of the health benefits and historical and cultural origins of this ancient art form
- Understand musical arrangements, instruments and costumes from ancient to modern times.

Neither will good teachers enforce their own personal influences on you as their learner.

When we begin to learn a practical or physical skill of any kind, which could be tennis or golf, playing the piano, singing, ballet or belly dancing, we are aiming at achieving some sort of 'skilled performance' which should be consistent, co-ordinated and smooth, and which finally, as we progress, becomes 'second nature'.

In moving gradually on from our very earliest attempts at these skills, to the skilled performance level, we go through four distinct phases:

1. *Unconscious incompetence* is when we are unaware of what we are doing wrong and how to put it right.
2. *Conscious incompetence* is when we have an awareness that we are getting some stage or stages of the activity wrong, but seem powerless to perform to the standard we are aiming at.
3. *Conscious competence* is when we get the whole concept right, but may have to concentrate very hard indeed to perfect our performance to obtain a professional standard.
4. *Unconscious competence* is when the performance is consistently accurate and smooth, and appears to be effortless.

When we begin to learn or teach a practical or physical skill, we are operating within the 'psychomotor domain' (pertaining to muscular activity associated with mental processes) which contains five levels of difficulty.

The five stages are:

1. *Naturalisation* – when you, the learner, have completed one or more skills with ease, and performance becomes automatic

2. *Articulation* – when you, the learner, can combine one or more skills in sequence with harmony and consistency
3. *Precision* – when you, the learner, can reproduce a skill with accuracy, proportion and exactness independently
4. *Manipulation* – when you, the learner, can perform the skill according to instruction rather than observation
5. *Imitation* – when you, the learner, observe the skill and try to repeat it.

When planning a lesson, a teacher should make the lesson objectives clear at the outset, have a clear beginning and ending, and work through a number of stages. He or she should also:

- Analyse the skill to be learned. This means breaking it down into its component parts, identifying the sequence of the activity and abilities needed.
- Assess you, the learner, as you may have had lessons elsewhere and picked up habits that need to be unlearned.
- Describe and demonstrate the movement so that you, the learner, acquire a clear visual picture of the skill and an understanding of why it is done in that particular way.

Practice and feedback is very important when teaching. One's job as a teacher is to observe, and to give you some feedback on your performance. If you are not doing it correctly then they should be able to identify what it is you are not doing correctly. Your teacher should remember to give affirmation that you are getting something right, praise you for your good effort, and encourage you to aspire to greater levels of performance.

It is so easy for a teacher to damage your confidence and self-esteem, and as a result you could easily become very frustrated and feel that you cannot achieve the goals you have been set, and that you are failing to progress to a level others have achieved. This is called 'hitting the plateau'; at this point it's important that your teacher exercises patience with you and takes time to devise the movement.

Sadly, I have received numerous complaints over the years about teachers and have selected some of the following situations, in which teachers:

- Have not covered the health and safety issues required
- Lack teaching skills and dance techniques
- Stand with their back to the learners throughout the session, looking in the mirror
- Do the movements and expect learners to follow what they are doing
- Make the class far too serious
- Create classes that are too cliquey
- Are biased and have favourites
- Ignore some learners
- Are condescending or make derogatory remarks
- Cannot break down and demonstrate a movement skilfully
- Refuse to demonstrate verbally, or non-verbally, a movement a second time when requested
- Are limited on the number of dance movements they can teach
- Cannot answer learners' questions on the history of the dance
- Lack knowledge of the health benefits of the dance
- Spend too much time talking instead of teaching
- Tend to teach more exercises than belly dance movements.

Some learners have even been told off for helping a fellow learner or for giggling in class, told to cover up their bare bellies or leave. I even received several reports about one particular teacher who apparently stamped her foot and told her learners that they would have to go round and round the room until they got a particular step right, even it took all night. Learners have come to me in tears after their teacher made the following remark to them: "I don't know why you're here – you'll never make a dancer." Such behaviour towards learners is unprofessional and unacceptable, and only serves to demonstrate their insecurity and incompetence within themselves as a teacher.

Dance classes should be inspirational, fun and relaxing. Making people laugh helps to break down barriers and is also therapeutic because it helps to improve your mood, relaxes you, makes you feel good and benefits your health. If your teacher is a good teacher he or she should have the ability to create a comfortable physical environment, a friendly atmosphere, and encourage learner participation. A class should also give learners the opportunity to make new friends.

A skilled teacher should be able to perform, demonstrate and break down a movement verbally and non-verbally, so that it will be clearly understood. If a teacher is conscientious, she/he will demonstrate a movement as many times as it is necessary. Patience is a virtue, and is what teaching is all about.

A teacher should be able to implement the best methods of analysis and instruction with patience, and have the ability to encourage learners, while recognising the need for critical analysis and definition.

Teachers should give every learner some individual attention during class, make sure that all members of the group are treated equally, and that there is an atmosphere of mutual respect between them and the members of the class. They should be able to make the subject interesting and structure learning so that learners leave with a sense of progress.

All teachers should be able to respond to anatomical, physio-logical and psychological problems with regard to improving your health and general well-being, which means: they should have some basic knowledge of common health problems, and be able to understand the health benefits to be gained from the movements of the belly dance, for example in pregnancy; the dance as a childbirth preparation; for back, hip and knee problems; IBS (irritable bowel syndrome) and digestive problems; poor posture, balance and co-ordination; and understand the meaning and complexities of dyspraxia. They should also be aware of learners who have poor eyesight or hearing problems, and those with the early stages of endometriosis, arthritis, multiple sclerosis, asthma, diabetes, epilepsy, tension and depression, cardiovascular disease and high blood pressure, and other health and fitness problems.

I remember one learner who attended one of my workshops who, after an hour into the session, looked rather pale and then became highly coloured. I asked her if she was OK; she said yes and told me she had a bit of a headache. I suggested she sat down for a while; she said she wanted to continue, but I insisted. She sat for a short while, then joined in again. Some time later I said, "Please sit down again", as I felt something wasn't right. But she was very persistent, saying she wasn't giving in – she was enjoying it too much. Later in the day I was so concerned about her I asked her not to do any more and to stay seated or go home, which made me feel awful. The following week she telephoned to say that she ended up in hospital that evening as an emergency with high blood pressure and was told she could have died. I shudder to think what would have happened if I had ignored her and not insisted she stopped dancing.

It is vitally important for a teacher to understand the implications of incorrect posture on one's health and how it can restrict one's ability to do the movements correctly, as well as recognising medical conditions such as scoliosis, lordosis, kyphosis, poor posture, balance and co-ordination, and knowing how to assess and help learners to overcome these particular problems through the dance.

One problem I come across frequently is the tendency for learners to turn either one or both of their feet in, particularly when travelling forward or doing steps on the spot such as the forward-step back-step. This can cause back problems and learners should be made aware of what they are doing, be encouraged not to turn their foot inwards, and be corrected whenever they do.

One learner did it so badly she ruined her shoes. Being encouraged to correct the foot helped her a great deal, so much in fact that she joined a circus training course and learnt to walk the tightrope.

Lack of confidence and low self-esteem are common problems among many women, therefore it is very important for a teacher to recognise those of you who are at a low ebb. There are numerous ways of helping to boost confidence and self-esteem: by encouraging you and others affected by these problems to become part of the group; praising your efforts; noting little things like one's change of hairstyle, loss of weight, or looking great in a costume; asking you, for example, how your back problem was after last week's class – did it feel better or did it feel worse?

Belly Dancing for Older Learners

For those of you in your sixties, seventies and even in your early eighties, belly dancing is an ideal form of exercise and great fun. As we get older many physiological changes arise and our general physical fitness level decreases. The loss of mobility is very much associated with the process of ageing and affects balance and co-ordination, which can result in falls.

Other risk factors are lack of flexibility and stamina, bone density, osteoporosis, postural changes, and gait abnormalities, which means the way you move when you walk, muscle weakness and poor strength; circulatory problems, high blood pressure and being prone to being overweight; a poor memory, lack of concentration; impaired vision and hearing problems.

I hasten to add there are many learners in their sixties who are very fit and healthy. Some of the problems I have mentioned can sometimes occur in people of a much younger age, so we cannot take it for granted that everyone over the age of 60 is unfit and has any of the problems associated with old age. But whatever your age, maintaining physical activity through the gentle movements of the belly dance will help to improve muscle tone, flexibility, stamina, balance and co-ordination. If you want to prevent premature ageing and dependence on others it is vitally important you take up some form of exercise, whether it be ballroom dancing, walking, swimming or belly dancing.

Safe and effective dance practice must be observed by all teachers to prevent any risk of injury to the participants. Ideally a teacher should have acquired a first-aid certificate and be able to render first-aid if and when needed, and must have liability insurance before starting to teach. So those of you who are thinking about joining a class, whatever your age or health and fitness levels, should not be afraid to ask the teacher if they are trained as a dancer, have done a teacher training course, etc., or have liability insurance, for if you injure yourself during a session you may not be able to claim any compensation. Here's an old saying that's worth remembering: "Teachers are born, not made."

Rhythm and Music

I think music in itself is healing. It's an explosive expression of humanity. It's something we are all touched by. No matter what culture we come from, everyone loves music.
(Billy Joel)

The perpetual motion of life is rhythm. Rhythm is life, the heartbeat of the universe, without which nothing could exist. Both humankind and the animal kingdom depend on the rhythm of life in order to survive, from the moment of conception and through life until death.

Our bodies constantly move in a rhythmic motion, and because of this natural creative force within us, regardless of whether or not we think we have no sense of rhythm, we unconsciously find ourselves drumming our fingers or tapping our feet when we hear a lively piece of music.

Dance is the language of life which, when accompanied by rhythm, awakens our inner responses, reflexes and motion within us, freeing us from lethargy and encouraging energy and vigour. Moving to rhythm allows our bodies to move instinctively, freeing our body, mind and spirit, gradually releasing an array of suppressed emotions. This not only enables us to express our sensuality, joy and sadness, but also shakes off all those unwanted inhibitions, breaking down the pattern of controlled behaviour that is expected of us during the course of our daily lives.

Dance movements performed today are rarely as expressive or as abandoned as those of our ancestors, apart from ancient tribal dances that have survived among modern primitive tribes in some remote areas of the world. The reason is that dance steps are precisely choreographed, and concentrated on the precise rhythm of the music, which tends to impede improvisation and the self-expression of the dancer.

Unfortunately many dance students and performers have copied routines which they have studied avidly from videos, or learnt from their teachers, which they then perform in a repetitive and unfeeling manner, completing the whole effect with a fixed smile. This alone is not enough. True art is spontaneous. A fixed smile is not only unattractive when performing, but also portrays the dancer's lack of depth, sincerity and emotion.

This unfeeling approach to any form of dance makes it virtually impossible for a student or performer to interpret and appreciate the various moods of the music with any emotion or self-expression.

Whatever medium of dance, be it ballet, tap, jazz or belly dancing, it is important for a dancer to be aware of his or her own body, and the art of moving their bodies in a spontaneous and rhythmic way.

A dancer's movements should be fluid, with each artistic movement flowing into another, interpreting the music through movement as the rhythm changes from a lively tempo, to a slow, dramatic or intense one, enabling the dancer to derive joy through the rhythm of music. This in turn helps the dancer to communicate with his or her inner self and portray various states of emotion and moods through the music.

It has always been assumed that we inherited the unity of dance and music from ancient human beings, who observed and imitated the animals and birds with their natural instinct for rhythm. Maybe they unconsciously linked their body movements to the rhythmic beat of their hearts, and the natural sounds of the Earth Mother, to accompany their animal, fertility and magic dances.

We can only imagine in our minds the rhythmic sounds they created to accompany their dance movements during such ritual dances. Originally, sounds were probably created vocally, or by clapping hands together, clicking their fingers, or slapping various parts of their bodies with their hands or elbows. Rhythmic sounds would also have been created by beating two sticks together, perhaps on a chunk of wood or stones, or created from rattles made of shells, wood, animal teeth, clay beads, ivory or bones that were either hand held or tied to some part of their bodies.

Whether learning to play a musical instrument, dancing or singing, one has to be able to understand rhythm. Rhythm is a grouping of beats, notes or measures which are an essential part of all music. Regular rhythmic beats can be produced by hand clapping, finger snapping, beating a drum or by playing other percussion instruments such as tambourines or cymbals. Rhythm is the flow that is created by the beat within the music.

Western music has a decisive regular rhythm and relies on a variety of changes in the tempo, which breaks down into 4/4, ¾¾ and 2/4 timing. Middle Eastern and North African rhythms, by contrast, cannot be divided evenly, as they are strung together in a series of smaller patterns which you may find rather difficult to understand at first. This is the essence of rhythm – our bodies moving to beats of the music and not the beats behind the music.

When you first begin to learn the dances of North Africa and the Middle East, you will have to listen to the music time and time again in order to gain some understanding of its complexities and the percussion instruments used, but with perseverance you will get used to the various beats and intricate rhythmic patterns that the music portrays.

You will also eventually recognise many of the percussion, wind and string instruments used. Having eventually accomplished an understanding of these complex rhythms, melodies and moods, you will able to interpret the mood and style of the music as you dance and become much more proficient as a dancer in this beautiful art form.

Although Middle Eastern music has definite rhythmic patterns, they are not always easy to follow. Eastern rhythms cannot be divided evenly, as they are strung together in a series of smaller patterns. The beat is defined by the DUM, the base beat, and the TAK, the light beat. In other words the down beat is the DUM and the up beat is the TAK. It may help you to understand if you try the following exercises.

Clap your hands together firmly, once to represent the down beat, DUM, then lightly clap your hands together once, to represent the TAK beat.

Now repeat the following sequences several times by clapping your hands together:

DUM – TAK, **DUM** – TAK, **DUM** – TAK, **DUM** – TAK

Now vary the rhythm by clapping your hands together firmly twice, then once lightly. It should sound like this:

DUM DUM – TAK, **DUM DUM** – TAK, **DUM DUM** – TAK, **DUM DUM** – TAK

Now try the following sequence:

DUM DUM TAK **DUM, DUM DUM** TAK **DUM, DUM DUM** TAK **DUM, DUM DUM** TAK **DUM**

Rhythms of Middle Eastern and North African music are many and varied, some being slow and stately, others fast and intricate. But anything else in between can be perceived as an arrangement of resonant dull strokes, traditionally taught aurally/orally from teacher to student.

In Turkey, finger snapping is also used as a rhythmic accompaniment for belly dancers instead of finger cymbals. I have tried and tried to snap my fingers rhythmically, but it's something that I have never been able to accomplish, much to my frustration, although many patient Middle Eastern musicians and dancers have tried to teach me.

To help you understand some of these complex rhythms, I have included a selection that are most commonly heard when learning to belly dance, which have been devised by that very talented Egyptian composer and percussionist, musician Hossam Ramzy, who has given me so much encouragement and inspiration.

- The *Fallahi* rhythm is played with two beats to the bar and used in songs of celebration by Egyptian peasant farmers, called the Fallaheen (a word from which the word Fallahi is derived).
- The *Masmoudi* rhythm is played in 8/4 time, eight beats to the bar. It has two parts of four counts following consecutively to make up the eight counts.
- Played in 4/4 time, four beats to the bar, is the *Ingara* or *Maqsoum*, a widely used Egyptian rhythm, which when played at a slower tempo makes another: *Masmoudi*.
- A 2/4 time rhythm that is usually played to accompany Oriental dancers as they enter and exit the stage is the *Malfuf* rhythm. It is also known as *Arabi,* which is a name not known in the West.
- A rhythm broadly used in Egyptian classical music is the *Sammaai* rhythm, which is a complex composition made up of a three-part sequence. The first part has three beats to the bar; the second, four beats to the bar; and the third part, three beats to the bar. When put together, these make a 10/8 rhythm.
- The *Elzaffa* rhythm is a wedding march in 4/4 time, played when accompanying dancers and sending the honeymooners on their way after the wedding celebrations.
- Other music which is commonly used to accompany dancers is the *Chifte-telli* or *Ciftitelli* and the *Baladi/Beledi.* The Ciftitelli is played in 4/4 time, has two parts and is also played in Turkish music. The Beledi is played at a slightly quicker tempo than the Ciftitelli. Traditionally the Beledi is a happy, lively dance of country folk and also means 'my people/village' or 'my country'.
- The *Karachi* rhythm is rather unusual as it starts with a *tak,* a treble beat, instead of the *dum* base beat, and has two

beats to the bar. Although the Karachi rhythm is not originally Egyptian, it is broadly used in Egyptian and North African music.

- A rhythm from Upper Egypt, used in a martial arts dance /combatic dance, which is performed by men wielding large heavy sticks, is the *Saaidi* rhythm, which is played with four beats to the bar.

- The *Kashlimar* is a 9/8 rhythm that originated from Turkey and was later adopted by the Greeks and used in folk dances.

- The haunting sounds of the *Taqsim*, or *Takseem* as it is sometime referred to, is traditionally an improvised solo piece of music played in a slow tempo. Usually it is played by one instrumentalist without any rhythmic percussion or singing accompaniment. That means that one does not have a regular beat to follow when dancing, which can be rather daunting for an inexperienced dancer. However, it does give a skilled performer an ideal opportunity to express personally this haunting mood of the music through his or her dance movements.

- ¾¾ time is also used in Egyptian music as in Western music.

To learn more, you can purchase *Introduction to Rhythms of the Nile* by Hossam Ramzy. Hossam's ever-increasing selection of Middle Eastern music is very popular with teachers, learners and performers and is available from most music stores. Visit www.Hossamramzy.com. Hossam is the owner of Drumzy Music Productions.

To give you an introduction to Middle Eastern dance music, I have chosen some CDs and certain tracks of music for you to practise your dance steps to, which should still be available in large music stores. You may also find them on the internet by just writing the name of the track into a search engine.

One collection of music I have not included is Mezdeke, *Sozlo-Pop Arabic / Misir Danslari* (Koda Muzik, 2005). There are a series of these tapes numbered 1 to 6 which are available in large music stores. It is great, lively music, excellent for hip bounces, hip twists and shimmies, and all learners enjoy dancing to it. For camel rocks, figure eights, hip swings and circles, I use track 1, 'Gani Lasmar', from Hossam Ramzy's *Egyptian Rai*.

Can Men Belly Dance?

Man learned to resort to dance when he felt helpless or fragmental and dislocated with the universe.
(Mary Austin, *The American Rhythm*, 1923)

Note: Some extracts from the following are mentioned in my previous book, *Belly Dance: The Dance of Mother Earth*.

The answer to the above question is yes, although the very concept of men belly dancing in the same manner of women is a very controversial subject among numerous women, who believe there is no place for male belly dancers. They are sincerely convinced that this art form was and still is originally for women, believing fervently that this ancient art form was and still is an empowerment of women, a powerful means through which they can celebrate and express their divine femininity. However, there are those who do believe that there is a place for men in Middle Eastern dance, especially in folkloric styles in authentic dress.

For centuries in Turkey, Egypt and Greece, men have played a special role in dance. In ancient times it was unusual for women to take part in secular, magical, phallic, hunting or war dances, as they were usually the only participants in fertility rituals, which consisted of birth dances, the consecration of young women, mourning rituals, sun and moon worship, rain and harvest dances. During the Ottoman Empire, dance evidence in the form of Turkish miniatures depicts young men called 'Koceks' who were employed by the Sultan to perform popular dances in preference to women who were prohibited from dancing. In the mid-1600s it's believed that there were approximately 3,000 of these dancers, divided into twelve companies. These female impersonators were young, effeminate, handsome boys highly trained in dance and music. Dressed in their wide flamboyant skirts, they performed acrobatics and sensuously shimmied, sashayed and undulated in a very provocative way. They rhythmically snapped their fingers or played wooden clappers which were eventually replaced by zills, small metal cymbals. They danced until the onset of puberty when they were no longer able to hide their whiskers.

During the era of Mahmud II in the 1800s the Koceks were officially banned from performing, which forced many to leave Turkey for Egypt and other countries. In Egypt young men called 'Khawals', mostly young men and boys who were Muslims and natives of Egypt, were hired to dance in preference to women. Mostly their dress consisted chiefly of a tight vest, a girdle and a type of petticoat. They imitated the female dancers by applying kohl to their eyes and henna to their feet, letting their hair grow long and braiding it in the manner of women. When in the streets and not engaged in dancing, they would often veil their faces to affect the manners of the women. The Khawals were frequently employed in preference to the Ghawazee gypsies to perform at popular festivals, to dance in front of a house or courtyard on the occasion of a marriage, birth or circumcision.

In Cairo there was another class of male dancer whose performances, dress and general appearance were similar to that of the Khawals. Generally they were Jews, Armenians, Greeks and Turks, though not of Egyptian blood. These female impersonators who danced in a similar style to that of the female dancers were distinguished by a different appellation, *gink*, a Turkish word that had a very vulgar significance. It is still common practice today for male dancers to imitate female dancers in some areas of Turkey; they are usually employed to perform at weddings and other celebrations.

A large majority of Middle Eastern men find male dancers who dance in the same manner as female dancers abhorrent and totally unacceptable. But they do accept males performing folkloric dances in traditional costumes at social functions and weddings, traditions that have survived for centuries in Egypt, Turkey and Morocco. In Egypt, in contrast to the undulating movements of the women, these masculine male dances involve much turning and leaping, often with the use of sticks or swords.

The upsurge of modern male belly dancing began in America in the 1960s and '70s, although it's become a very debatable topic among the female belly dance fraternity. There are many well-known male performers and teachers, including Khalid, Horatio and Ozgen, and it's something we will have to accept, whatever our opinions, as I believe they are here to stay.

So, if men do take up belly dancing, will they gain the same health benefits as women? Yes, in some ways they will. It's a good abs and cardiovascular workout, and will help those with low back pain, loosen stiff joints, tone flabby muscles, and improve posture, poor co-ordination and balance.

Since the 1970s men have joined my classes for several reasons, and before you shake your hands in horror, under the Sex Discrimination Act one is obliged to let them join a class; it would now be a problem trying to bar them.

I have to admit that I have had a couple of problems with voyeurs and some absolute nuts, who for the safety of my learners and myself had to be dealt with promptly. But over the years I have had several really nice guys who have come along with their girlfriends or wives for a workout and thoroughly enjoyed the session. For at least two years a medical doctor came along with his wife and 3-year-old son. When his wife became pregnant they continued classes until it was almost time for her to give birth. Two weeks after the birth they were back in class with the baby in a carry cot. This doctor was extremely supportive of the belly dance, not only as an excellent exercise for pregnant women, but also as a great exercise to improve one's health and general well-being.

One guy, a martial arts expert, told me that the belly dancing was great for improving his balance, stamina and co-ordination, but he made me promise I would never tell his wife that he came along to my classes. Other men came, claiming it helped to improve their skiing and martial arts, while others said it definitely improved their low back pain, and boosted their energy levels.

I will always remember one guy (married) who turned up for one of my workshops in London, wearing nothing more than a leather thong. You can imagine the expressions on the faces of the women; they were an absolute picture. They just could not believe what they were seeing and to be honest nor could I. Some of the group were very embarrassed and one or two said that he should not be allowed to take part in the workshop. Luckily the majority just burst into fits of giggles, commenting that in no way would they be able to stand behind him while he was practising the movements! After I had a quiet word with him, he realised his folly and covered up, and being such a really nice, unassuming, charming guy, he quickly won the women round. I'm happy to say that after attending his very first workshop he continued to attend my evening classes and those of other teachers and eventually became an accomplished performer.

So yes, rightly or wrongly I would confirm that men can belly dance!

(Sources: Tina Hobin, *Belly Dancing for Health and Relaxation*, Duckworths; *Belly Dance: The Dance of Mother Earth*, published by Marion Boyars; Metin And, *A Pictorial History of Turkish Dance*, Musikgeschichte in Bildern, UNESCO, Kommission der DDR, 1983)

The Ancient Art of the Belly Dance

This wondrous miracle did love devise,
For dancing is love's proper exercise.
(John Davies, 1569–1626)

The Belly Dance

Ideally, belly dancing classes where training can be given by an expert are the best places to learn. The group atmosphere provides companionship and plenty of fun, as well as speeding the learning process. However, for various reasons not every enthusiast can attend classes, but it is quite possible for anyone to learn at home from this book, if the step-by-step guide and detailed instructions are followed carefully.

The following dance steps have been designed systematically to follow in sequence, each one leading naturally to the next. In this step-by-step guide on how to belly dance the movements are gentle to begin with, and will allow your body to adjust and warm up without any undue stress or strain. Be sensible and limit your practice sessions at first, particularly if you haven't exercised or danced for some time or have had an illness or injury.

Note: Remember, stretching exercises should *not* be used as warm-ups as they could result in stressing and straining which will damage your muscles, tendons and ligaments. So please refer to the warm-up section on page 71.

When practising, choose a room that is airy and has plenty of space. Remove any loose rugs and furniture that has sharp corners such as a coffee table.

If you have polished wooden floors or tiled floors, do not wear socks or tights as you may slip and have a nasty fall. Wear either soft flexible shoes or practise in your bare feet.

To ensure you are doing the movements correctly, a full-length mirror is an asset but not a necessity. A smaller mirror can be used to observe your hips and abdomen as long as it is positioned safely.

To allow freedom of movement when doing the belly dance movements, do not wear clothes that are restricting like tight jeans or skirts. Wear light, loose clothing such as baggy trousers, leggings, or a skirt with an elasticised waist, so that it can be pulled down and worn around the hips. For the top half, wear a bikini top, bra or a blouse you can tie under the midriff.

Many doctors, physiotherapists, chiropractors and osteopaths are now aware of the health benefits of the belly dance, and may recommend that you attend a class to help alleviate your particular problem. However, if your tutor has not approached you and asked you about your medical condition you must make a point of informing him or her. It is vitally important that you are advised correctly on what movements you should or should not do, as some may aggravate your problem. And please, if you are asked if you do have a medical problem, declare it. I get rather annoyed when a learner declines to tell me after being asked, only to be told some weeks later that they do have a particular medical problem.

Dos and don'ts

Many teachers and learners tend to favour using one side more than the other when dancing. If you do most of the movements on one side only, it will eventually become overdeveloped, and as a result, the muscles on the less favoured side will become weaker, and the joints stiffer and less mobile, which is not good for balance, posture and perfect muscle development. However difficult it may be for some of you, it is important to exercise both sides equally, so do persevere. And please at all times remember the breathing techniques and inhale and exhale gently through your nose.

Correct starting position

Before commencing a dance movement you should be instructed to assume the correct starting position.

- Drop shoulders down and lift head up.
- Stand with your feet apart at hip width or as instructed.
- Elevate rib cage, i.e. lift rib cage.
- Knees flexed, i.e. bend them very slightly.
- Hold both feet firmly to the floor.

Remember to keep your weight evenly distributed when both feet are firmly on the floor, when you place one foot forward or rise up onto the balls of both feet.

- Do not turn your toes up or roll onto the outside or inside of your feet.
- Do not turn your foot inwards when placing the foot forward.
- Do not swing your knee out when pushing the hip out.
- Do not lock your knees.
- Do not dance with knees bent too much.
- Do not lean back.

And observe the breathing techniques.

Note: To refresh your memory on the importance of these specific points, please refer to pages 68–70.

Arm movements

When practising arm movements, poor co-ordination and lack of awareness of perception can be a problem. For example, when you're asked to place your right hand on your temple, you will have placed it anywhere but on your temple. And when asked to raise your arm up straight above your head, it ends up bent at the elbow, held across your face, dropped to the side of your head or out to the side. So, when practising your arm and hand movements, stand in front of a full-length or half-sized mirror which is big enough to see your arms when extended above your head or held out to the sides.

Hands and arms play an important role in dance, and must never be neglected. Don't hold them with elbows locked, drop them down lifelessly at your sides, clench your fists or hold your fingers stiffly, as that is an indication of tension or stress. Hand movements should be gentle and supple, with fingers relaxed.

The soft, flowing and snake-like movements of the hands and arms should at all times complement and enhance the line of your body movements. Practising the arm movements will also strengthen your upper arms and upper body.

There is also a common tendency for some teachers and dancers to continually rotate their hands when dancing; this can be very annoying, and distracts from the dance movements.

When learning the movements of the belly dance for the first time, you may find that using your arms at the same time as doing a movement may be a little difficult, as it's like patting your head and rubbing your tummy at the same time. So start with your arms down at your side, then raise them up no higher than waist level and take them out slightly to the side so that your elbows are level with your waist. When you feel confident with the movements, then you can start to introduce the arms.

If you get a stitch when practising the exercises or dance steps, stop and try the following:

1. Stand with your feet slightly apart.
2. Elevate your rib cage.
3. Place both arms down by your side.
4. As you inhale, slowly raise both arms until above your head, placing hands back to back.
5. Lower both arms to shoulder level.
6. Repeat twice more, then lower your arms down to your

sides.

Your stitch should have now eased or gone.

Arms

- When held out to the side the arms should be no higher than shoulder level with elbows relaxed.
- Arms should be held below bust level when out in front of you.
- When held slightly out to the sides, elbows should be at waist level.
- When held down by your side, arms should be rounded at the elbow to frame your hip.
- When raised above your head, they should be rounded at the elbow with hands pointing towards each other or pointing up towards the ceiling with the hands placed back to back.
- When you raise one arm up above your head, do not neglect the other arm; all too often it just hangs down totally forgotten.

Don't forget to do some gentle arm movements to warm up before you begin, then follow with the hip rotations.

Hip Rotations

Music for hip rotations

Burhan Ocol, Istanbul Oriental Ensemble, *Gypsy Rum*
Track 8: 'Hicazkar Sahin Oyun Havasi'

Solace, *Rhythm of the Dance* (Eventide Music Productions)
Track 1: 'Beledi'

Fat Chance Belly Dance, Helm, *Tribal Dance, Tribal Drums*
Track 1: 'Maqsoum'

Track 4: 'Moroccan 6'

The following movements are either described as hip circles or hip rotations.

a) Assume starting position.
b) When doing hip rotations/circles, your knees should always be slightly flexed and held steady. Do not move them.
c) Stand with your feet apart at hip width, and weight even on both feet.
d) Hold your arms out to the side, palms facing either up or down.
e) Stick your bottom out and roll your hips over to the right side, then...
f) Push your pelvis forward as far as you can and roll the hips over to the left.
g) Push your pelvis back to the rear (in other words, stick your bottom out), then immediately roll your hips over to the right.
h) Push the pelvis forward again and continue to rotate your hips smoothly in a large circle several times.
i) Repeat the movement by rotating your hips in the opposite direction several times.

Note: I always tell my students: the bigger the bum, the better for belly dancing, so use it!

Variation 1 on the hip circle

a) Rotate your hips in a circle in one direction twice.
b) Then rotate the hips twice in the opposite direction.
c) Repeat this movement several times, rotating your hips twice in one direction, then twice in the opposite direction.

Variation 2 on the hip circle

a) Rotate your hips, making one very large, smooth circle.

b) Follow the large rotation with two smaller rotations in the same direction.

Repeat this movement several times in one direction and then in the opposite direction.

Arm movements with hip rotations

a) Start by placing your arms down by your side.

b) Bring them forward and up a little, then take them out slightly to the side so that your elbows are level with your waist.

c) As you circle your hips, bring your arms forward until your hands touch back to back just below belly button level.

d) While continuing to circle your hips, gently take your arms back and cross your hands just below the cheeks of your bottom.

Small hip circles

a) Stand with your feet close together but not touching.

b) Flex your knees and hold your feet firmly to the floor.

c) Elevate your rib cage.

d) Hold your arms slightly out to the side with elbows at waist level.

e) Rotate your hips in a small circular motion several times to the right, and then several times to the left.

Arm position for small hip circles and alternate side hip circles

a) Place your arms down by your side.

b) Bring them forward until your elbows are at waist level.

c) Move them slightly out to the side. Hold them steady in

this position while doing the small hip rotation.

Pivoting hip circles with arms

Music

Slow or medium tempos are used for hip rotations.

Assume starting position.
   a) Hold your right arm out to the front and relax your elbow.
   b) Hold your left arm out to the side just below shoulder level and relax the elbow.
   c) Place your right leg directly forward with heel raised and knee slightly bent.
   d) Flex the left knee.
   e) Circle your right hip, as you pivot to the left on the flat of your left foot.

You should be able to do six hip circles as you pivot around on the spot, back to your starting position.

Change feet and the position of your arms so that your left arm is forward and your right one out to the side. Do six circles with your left hip as you pivot to the right on the flat of the right foot.

Hip circle with hip drop

This is a gentle movement done to a slow or medium tempo.

Music

Solace, *Rhythm of the Dance*
Track 1: 'Beledi'
Track 4: 'Beledi'(4)
Track 2: 'Chifte-telli'

Assume starting position.
   a) Hold arms out to the side just below shoulder level and relax the elbows.
   b) Stand with feet apart no wider than your hip line.
   c) Keeping your feet apart and parallel, raise your right heel and hip, then circle your hips anti-clockwise.
   d) Simultaneously lower the right heel, raise your left heel and hip, then circle your left hip clockwise.
   e) Simultaneously lower your left heel, raise your right heel and drop your right hip. (Footwork should be a smooth rock from one foot to the other.)
   Repeat the combination several times.

Pelvic roll

Music for pelvic roll

Hossam Ramzy, *Baladi Plus*
Track 6: 'Wahda We Bas'

Solace, *Rhythm of the Dance*
Track 1: 'Beledi'

Assume starting position.
   a) Rib cage elevated.
   b) Stand with your feet apart as wide as your hip line.
   c) Weight evenly distributed on both feet, flex knees and hold steady.
   d) Place arms up and out to the side just below shoulder level and elbows relaxed.
   e) Stick your bottom out as far as you can and slowly roll your pelvis over to the right, making an arc, and then straighten up. (When doing the hip roll, the further you push your hips back, the more you will be tempted to lean forward too much. You should only lean forward slightly.)

f) Stick your bottom out again and slowly roll your pelvis over to the left, making an arc, then straighten up.

Repeat several times, pushing your bottom out as far as you can and rolling your pelvis from right to left in a smooth, continuous motion.

Forward hip roll

a) Push your pelvis forward and roll your hips from right to left, making an arc.
b) Then, roll your pelvis from left to right. Imagine you are only doing half a hip rotation.
c) Repeat the movement by smoothly rolling your hips from left to right, then right to left. Repeat several times.
Now try the same movement using the feet.

Pelvic hip roll with footwork

Assume starting position.
a) Stand with your feet apart at hip width.
b) As soon as you begin to roll your pelvis over to the left, raise your right heel.
c) When you have rolled your pelvis over to the left, lower the right heel.
d) As soon as you begin to roll your pelvis over to the right, raise your left heel.
e) Repeat the movement several times.

Pelvic roll with hip circle

a) Assume starting position.
b) Stand with feet apart no wider than your hip line and held firmly to the floor with your weight evenly distributed.
c) Push your bottom out and roll your hips from left to right very slowly. It is usually done to six or eight counts depending on the music.

d) From this position (right) push your bottom out and roll over to the left and immediately push forward to complete a hip rotation.

e) Repeat the movement, pushing your bottom out from the right and rolling your pelvis slowly over to the left.

f) From this position (left) push your bottom out, roll over to the right, then do a complete hip rotation.

Double roll and hip circle

a) Assume starting position.

b) Feet apart as wide as your hip line and held firmly to the floor with your weight evenly distributed.

c) Push your pelvis forward, then roll your hips from right to left, then left to right, right to left, and follow with a large hip circle.

Repeat several times.

Step pattern

It may make it easier to repeat to yourself as you do the movement:

Roll – roll – roll and circle, roll – roll – roll and circle, roll – roll – roll and circle

Now try the movement rolling your hips out to the rear, from right to left, left to right, and follow with a circle.

Arm movement

a) Place your arms down by your side.

b) Raise them out to the side.

c) Relax the elbows which should be held at waist level.

Basic right and left hip circles

Music for hip circles

Hossam Ramzy, *Source of Fire*
Track 2: 'Manbaa Innar'

Fat Chance Belly Dance, Helm, *Tribal Dance, Tribal Drums*
Track 1: 'Maqsoum'
Track 11: 'Baladi'

Solace, *Rhythm of the Dance*
Track 2: 'Chifte-telli'
Track 4: 'Beledi'

When doing these circles, don't place your leg too far out; if you do, it is more difficult to do a proper circle of the hips. Don't straighten your knee or swing the knee out to the side. Keep your heel up, knee bent, and hold your knee steady over your foot.

a) Assume starting position.
b) Stand with your feet close together but not touching, with weight evenly distributed.
c) Place your right leg forward.
d) Raise your right heel, bend your right knee and keep your left knee flexed.
e) While keeping the right heel up and the knee bent, rotate your right hip anti-clockwise in a smooth circle.
Repeat several times.

Now circle your right hip in the opposite direction, pushing your hip back. When pushing the hip back, do not swing your knee out to the side.
Repeat several times.

a) Place your left leg forward.
b) Raise your left heel, bend your left knee, flex your right knee.

c) Rotate your left hip in a smooth circle anti-clockwise several times.

d) Repeat the movement by rotating the hip in the opposite direction, pushing your hip back.

Repeat several times, and watch those knees.

Right and left hip rotation variations

Assume the same position as with the basic hip rotation by placing the right leg forward, raising the heel of the right leg and flexing the left knee. This movement consists of one large hip rotation followed by two undulating hip rotations.

Now try this undulating variation:

a) Assume the same starting position.

b) Place the right leg forward and raise the heel and keep the heel raised throughout the movement.

c) Flex the left knee.

d) Slowly do a large circle with your right hip anti-clockwise.

e) As you bend both knees, do two smaller and slightly quicker circles in the same direction.

f) Come up slowly and smoothly.

g) Repeat this movement several times, then repeat on the left side. Remember to keep your back straight as you bend your knees.

Repeat several times, then do the movement on the left side, circling the hip clockwise.

Arm movement

a) If you place your right leg forward, raise your left arm up and bend it gently so that the arm is curved above your head.

b) Hold your right arm down by your side and round it at the elbow, so that your arm is softly framing your hip and the hand is gently pointing towards your right hip.

When you place your left leg forward, reposition your

arms by raising the right arm up and gently bend it so that the arm is curved above your head and the left one is down, framing the left hip.

Circle within a circle

Music for circle within circles and combinations
Hossam Ramzy, *Best of Abdul Halim Hafiz*
Side B, Track 1: 'Ganalhawa' (on cassette)

You may find this particular movement a bit difficult to do at first. But if you follow the instructions carefully, you will soon master it.

Your feet must be kept flat on the floor and apart at hip width. It is also important to keep your feet parallel throughout the movement. If you place one foot slightly further forward than the other, your hips will twist as you circle.

Warning: This movement is not advisable if you suffer from low back pain as the back hyper-extends and may aggravate your problem. But when your back feels stronger do give it a go, as it is a very graceful movement.

a) Assume starting position.
b) Stand with your feet apart as wide as your hips.
c) Flex both your knees.
d) Practise the basic step first.
e) Keeping your feet parallel, take a very tiny step forward onto the flat of the right foot, and as you do so, pivot slightly on the flat of your left foot to the left.
f) Continue stepping onto the flat of the right foot until you have completed a full circle on the spot and are back to the starting position.

Now try this step with the hip circle:

a) As you step onto the flat of the right foot, push your bottom out to the rear and complete a large hip circle from right to left (anti-clockwise) as you pivot very slightly on the flat of your left foot to the left.

b) Immediately take another tiny step onto the flat of the right foot and, as you do so, push your pelvis to the rear, and complete another hip circle from right to left (anti-clockwise) as you pivot very slightly to the left on the flat of your left foot.

c) Continue to pivot on your left foot, turning to the left as you circle your hips.

Now try this movement in the opposite direction:

a) As you step onto the flat of the left foot, push your pelvis to the rear and circle your hips from left to right (clockwise) as you pivot on the flat of the right foot to the right.

b) Continue to pivot on your right foot to the right, as you circle your hips.

Pelvic Tilts

Music for pelvic tilts
Hossam Ramzy, *Best of Mohammed Abdul Wahab*
Track 3: 'Khai Khai'

This movement is a gentle rocking of the pelvis to and fro. It must not be thrust to and fro aggressively. It is a great movement for helping to ease low back pain and stretching and strengthening the pelvic floor. This is also a good exercise to do if you are pregnant or have digestive or gynaecological problems.

a) Assume starting position.
b) Stand with your feet slightly apart and knees flexed.
c) Hold your knees steady. Do not move them to and fro when doing this movement.
d) Push your pelvis back (i.e. stick out your bottom out), then immediately thrust the pelvis forward and tilt upwards.

e) Push your pelvis back again, then immediately thrust the pelvis forward and tilt upwards.
Repeat the movement several times.

Undulating pelvic tilt

a) Tilt your pelvis to and fro four times as you bend both your knees, then to and fro four times as you come up until your knees are slightly bent.
b) Repeat several times.
Remember to keep your back straight as you bend your knees and do not lock the knees when you come up; keep them flexed.

Travelling pelvic tilt

a) Assume starting position.
b) As you take a very short step forward onto the flat of the right foot, tilt your pelvis forward back, forward back.
c) Then take a short step forward onto the flat of your left foot and tilt your pelvis forward back, forward back.
d) Continue tilting your pelvis to and fro as you take small alternative steps forward on the right then left foot.
Now try the movement stepping backwards. With practice you should be able to do this movement quickly.

Arms for pelvic tilt

a) Place your arms down by your side.
b) Raise them up in front of you no higher than the bust line.
c) Relax the elbows, and raise your hands.
d) As you do your pelvic tilts, roll your hands outwards until the palms of your hands face upwards, then inwards until the palms of your hands face the floor.

Basic Hip Drops and Bounces

A drop is when you drop the hip once. A bounce is when you

drop the hip more than once, i.e. at least twice or more times consecutively.

Music for hip drops and bounces
Chalf Hassan, *Belly Dance from Morocco*
Track 5: 'Solo Darbuka'

Solace, *Rhythm of the Dance*
Track 5: 'Saidi'

a) Assume starting position.
b) Stand with your feet close together but not touching, and flex knees.
c) Raise your right heel and bend your right knee.
d) Keep your left knee flexed throughout the movement. Do not lock the knee or move the knee to and fro.
e) Push your right hip down towards the floor, then raise it up till level.
f) Continue to drop and raise your hip to the rhythm of the music.

Step pattern
It may help if you repeat to yourself as you do the movement:
Down Up, Down Up, Down Up, Down Up, Down Up, Down Up
Repeat the movement on your left side.

If you find the hip drops a little difficult to do, place your hands on your hips and push your right hip down with your right hand. Then do the same on the left side.

Hip bounce variation
a) Assume starting position.
b) Stand with your feet slightly apart.
c) Raise your right heel, bend your right knee.

d) Keep your left knee flexed throughout the movement; do not lock the knees or move the knees to and fro.

You may find it difficult to drop your hips after pushing the hips back, so only take the hip back as far as you can comfortably. Do not force the hip back until you have loosened up.

a) Twist your right hip forward.
b) Drop and raise the hip twice, i.e. Down Up, Down Up.
c) Push the hip back, then drop and raise the hip twice, i.e. Down Up, Down Up.
d) Continue the movement several times, then try it on the left side.

Now try the single hip drop, forward and back.

Hip bounce variation

Assume starting position.

a) Turn your body so that you are facing side on.
b) Keep your right foot flat on the floor.
c) Take your left leg back, relax the knee and raise the heel.
d) Now turn your upper torso slightly towards the front.
e) Bounce your left hip several times.

Now try the movement on your right side.

a) Turn to the left so that you are facing side on.
b) Keep your left foot flat and knee flexed.
c) Take your right leg back, relax the knee.
d) Turn your upper torso slightly towards the front.
e) Bounce your right hip several times.

Variation

When you have mastered that movement, bend both knees as you bounce your hip four times, then bounce your hip four times as you rise up. Repeat several times on the left hip, then on the right hip.

Hip bounce combinations

a) Assume starting position.
b) Stand with your feet slightly apart.
c) Raise your right heel, bend the right knee. Flex the left knee.
d) Push your hip down twice: bounce bounce.
e) Twist hip forward and drop the hip once.
f) Push back and drop the hip once.
g) Twist your hip forward and drop again.
   Repeat several times.

Dance step pattern

Bounce bounce – forward drop – back drop – forward drop
Repeat the sequence, starting with the double bounce.

Practise this movement on your right side until you get into a rhythm, and then try it on your left side.

Variation on hip drops

a) Assume starting position.
b) Stand with your feet apart as wide as your hip line.
c) Keep your feet parallel throughout the movement and flex knees.
d) Raise your right heel and bounce your right hip down twice.
e) As you lower your right heel, raise your left heel and drop your left hip once.

Pattern

Right hip – bounce~bounce – left hip – drop
Repeat the sequence several times.

Then do two bounces on your left hip, then one on your right hip. Repeat the sequence several times.

When you have mastered the movement on the spot, try turning to the left. Start with the two bounces on your right hip, then one drop on your left hip and take a very, very tiny step forward on the right foot and do the two bounces on the right hip, then a hip drop on the left hip.

Repeat until you are back at your starting position, then do the movement turning to the right, starting with the two bounces on your left hip and one on your right hip.

Arm movements
Use the same arm movements as you did for the pelvic tilt. Or hold your arms out to the side below shoulder level with elbows relaxed.

Variation on hip bounces
When taking the hips back do not swing your knee outward; the knee should be held steady over the foot throughout the movement.

a) Assume starting position.
b) Stand with your feet slightly apart
c) Place your right leg forward, but not too far forward as this will prevent you from relaxing the knee; raise the heel.
d) Do four hip bounces as you push the hip back, and four hip bounces as you bring the hip forward. Repeat several times.
e) Place your left leg forward and bounce your left hip back four times, then four times as you bring your hip forward. Repeat several times.

Dance step pattern
Count as you drop your hips:
Back 1 2 3 4, Forward 1 2 3 4

Arm movement
a) If starting the movement with your right hip, raise your right arm forward below shoulder level and relax the

elbow.

b) Hold your left arm out to the left and bend it at the elbow.

c) As you drop your right hip back, slowly take your right arm back, then bring it forward as you bring your hips forward.

Change arms when you change feet or hold your arms in the same position, but don't take the arm back and forward as you bounce your hips back and forward.

Alternate hip drops

Music for hip drops
Use the tracks you played for the previous hip drops, plus:

Hossam Ramzy, *Best of Abdul Halim Hafiz*
Track 2: 'Khusara Khusara'

a) Stand with your feet close together but not touching.

b) Bend both your knees and hold them steady. It is very tempting to move the knees while doing this movement, but if you move your knees around or move them to and fro it will make the movement jerky, and certainly will not help your knees.

c) Place your hands on your hips.

d) Push down your hips alternatively.

When you have mastered this basic hip drop, with practice you will eventually be able to do it quite quickly which is how it should be done. When you can shimmy, do the alternate hip drops with the shimmy – it's a very effective movement!

Variation on hip drops
Instead of doing one hip drop on the right, then one on the left, try doing two hip drops on the right, then two on the left, to a

count of "1, 2".

Right hip: 1 2. Then left hip: 1 2.

Arm movement

Raise both arms up above your head, then drop them at the elbows; keep the hands up and hold this position throughout the movement. To vary the arm movement, rotate both your hands to the count of "1, 2", so that the hands face inwards on the count of 1, and outwards on the count of 2.

Basic Pivoting Hip Thrust

Music for all pivoting hip movements
Hossam Ramzy, *Best of Mohammed Abdul Wahab*
Track 2: 'Set Elhabayib Ya Habiba'

It's very tempting when doing this movement to lean to the left when pivoting to the left and when pivoting to the right lean to the right, or lean back slightly, so please follow the instructions correctly. Practise the basic movement first.
a) Assume starting position.
b) Stand with your feet close together but not touching.
c) Place your right leg forward and raise the heel.
d) Make sure your weight is evenly distributed on both feet.
e) Flex your left knee.
Practise the basic movement first by raising and lowering the ball of the foot to the floor. Now, as you lower the ball of the foot to the floor, push your hip out and up. Repeat several times, then practise this on your left side.
Now try it with the pivot:
a) Raise your right foot slightly off the floor, then, as you lower the ball of the foot to the floor, push your right hip out and up as you pivot a little to the left.

b) Immediately raise the ball of the right foot again, and as you lower the ball of the foot to the floor, push your right hip out and pivot a little to your left.

Repeat several times until back at your starting position.

Then practise the movement turning in the opposite direction:

a) Place your left leg forward with heel raised.

b) Raise your left foot slightly off the floor, then, as you lower the ball of the foot to the floor, push your left hip out and up as you pivot a little to the right.

c) Immediately raise the ball of the foot again and as you lower the ball of the foot to the floor, push your left hip out as you pivot to the right.

Repeat several times until back at your starting position.

If your back is strong and flexible, and back bends are not a problem, you can do the pivoting movement while arching back. But please do not attempt this if you have any back problems, no matter how slight.

Pivoting double hip thrust

Music for pivoting hip steps
Hossam Ramzy, *Best of Mohammed Abdul Wahab*
Track 2: 'Set Elhabayib Ya Habiba'

Richard Hagopian, Omar Faruk Tekbilek, *Gypsy Fire*
Track 3: 'Istemem Babacim'

This step is basically the same as the previous pivoting hip thrust, but this time you do a double hip push.

Assume starting position. Feet close together but not touching. Weight evenly distributed.

a) Place your right foot directly forward and raise the heel.

b) Keep your left foot flat on the floor and flex knee.

c) Raise the ball of the right foot up slightly off the floor, then...

d) Lower the ball of the right foot to the floor, and hold it to the floor as you push your right hip out and up twice to a quick count of "1, 2", then pivot a little to the left on the flat of the left foot.

e) Raise and lower the ball of the right foot again, hold it to the floor as you push your right hip up and out twice, then pivot a little to the left on the flat of the left foot.

f) Repeat the double hip push to the left several times until back at your starting position.

Now practise the movement pivoting to the right, by placing your left leg forward with the heel raised, and doing the double hip push with the left hip and pivot to the right on the flat of the right foot.

Pivoting hip bounce

Assume starting position. Feet close together. Weight evenly distributed.

Practise this on the spot first.

a) Raise your right heel and bend the right knee.

b) Flex your left knee.

c) Place your right hand on your right hip.

d) Raise your right foot very slightly off the floor.

e) As you lower the ball of the foot to the floor, push your right hip down with your right hand, then immediately lift up your right hip.

Repeat this several times, pushing the hip down, then lifting the hip up; then practise the movement on your left side.

Now combine the hip drop with the pivot:

a) Raise the right heel.

b) Push your right hip down, then immediately lift your right hip up as you pivot slightly to the left on the flat of your left foot.

c) Continue to pivot to the left until back at your starting position.

Repeat the movement several times on the left hip as you pivot to the right.

Double pivoting hip bounce

a) When you have mastered the single pivoting hip drop, try the pivoting hip bounce by dropping the right hip down twice in quick succession.

b) Continue the movement several times, pivoting to the left on the flat of the left foot, then change feet and bounce the left hip twice as you pivot to the right, on the flat of the right foot.

Step pattern

Count "1, 2" as you do the double bounce:

1 2 – 1 2 – 1 2 – 1 2

bounce bounce – bounce bounce – bounce bounce – bounce bounce

Double pivoting hip bounce with hip twist

This movement is the same as the pivoting double hip bounce, but this time you add two extra hip bounces.

a) Assume starting position.

b) Stand with your feet close together.

c) Raise your right heel.

d) Flex your left knee.

e) As you pivot to the left, simultaneously twist your right hip forward and bounce your hip twice.

f) Keeping the ball of the foot on the floor, immediately push the hip back and bounce your right hip twice.

g) Continue to pivot to the left as you twist your right hip forward and bounce it twice, then push it back and bounce it twice.

Repeat the movement several times as you turn to the left.

a) Change feet and raise your left heel.

b) Pivot to the right as you twist your left hip forward and bounce the hip twice, push the left hip back and bounce the hip twice.

Repeat several times as you turn to the right.

Dance step pattern

Twist hip forward and bounce~bounce
Push hip back and bounce~bounce

Pivoting undulating double hip bounce

Assume starting position.

a) Raise your right heel, flex left knee.

b) As you pivot to the left, raise and lower the ball of the right foot and do a double hip bounce, immediately raise the ball of the foot again, and as you lower it to the floor, bend both knees and bounce your right hip twice.

c) Continue to bounce your hips, doing two when upright, then two down, with both knees bent as you pivot to the left on the flat of the left foot.

Repeat the movement pivoting to the right, then repeat it to the left. Remember to keep your back straight when you bend your knees.

Pivoting hip bounces with turn

Assume starting position.

a) Stand with feet close together but not touching.

b) Raise your right heel.

c) Flex your left knee.

d) Depending on the music, do two or three double hip bounces, turning to the left on the flat of your left foot.

e) Keeping the right leg close to the floor, swing the leg

forward and over to the left. This movement of the right leg will help spin you round to face the front again.

f) Both feet should now be flat on the floor.

g) Raise your left heel and do three pivoting hip bounces turning to the right.

h) Keeping your left leg close to the floor, swing the leg forward and over to the right. You should have completed the turn and now be facing the front again.

Instead of doing hip bounces, do hip pushes. The number of bounces you do depends on the rhythm and beat of the music as you may have to do two or four hip bounces.

Four double hip bounces on the spot

a) Assume starting position.

b) Feet close together but not touching.

c) Place your right foot forward.

d) Raise the heel and flex the knee and bounce your hip twice.

e) Keeping the heel raised, take your right leg back until it is behind you and bounce your hip twice.

f) Bring the right leg forward and bounce your hip twice.

g) Take the right leg back and bounce your hip twice.

Repeat the sequence several times, then repeat on your left side.

Four double hip bounces turning on the spot

a) Assume starting position.

b) Stand with feet close together.

c) Place your right leg forward with heel raised and flex the knee.

d) Flex the left knee.

e) Bounce your right hip twice.

f) Take the right leg out behind you and bounce the hip twice.

g) Pivot slightly to the left.

h) Bring the right leg forward and do another double bounce.

i) Take the leg back and do another double bounce as you continue to pivot to the left.

Repeat until back at your starting position.

a) Place your left leg forward and do a double bounce.

b) Take your left leg back and do a double bounce.

c) Pivot slightly to the right and continue until back at your starting position.

Now try doing it in quarter turns.

Step: hip bounce variation

Face the left-hand corner.

a) Assume starting position.

b) Stand with feet close together but not touching.

c) Place your right leg forward with the heel raised and do a double bounce.

d) Take the right leg back until it is behind you and do a double bounce.

e) Place the right leg forward again and do a double bounce.

f) Take the right leg back again and do another double bounce.

g) Bring the right leg forward again and do four bounces while pushing the hip back and do four bounces as you bring the hip forward.

Repeat several times.

Now face the right-hand corner.

a) Place your left leg forward with heel raised and do two bounces.

b) Take the leg back and do two double hip bounces.

c) Bring the leg forward and do two hip bounces.

d) Take the leg back and do two hip bounces.

e) Bring the leg forward and do four hip bounces while pushing the hip back and four bounces as you bring the hip forward.

Repeat the sequence.

Arms for the hip bounce sequence

Place your right arm out to the right just below shoulder level with elbow relaxed. Place your left arm forward just below shoulder level and relax elbow.

Forward-Step Back-Step

(Kashlimar)

Music for forward-step back-steps

Various Artists, *Best of Bellydance from Morocco, Egypt, Lebanon, Turkey* (Arc Music)

Track 1: Hossam Ramzy & His Egyptian Ensemble, 'Enta Omri'

Solace, *Rhythm of the Dance*
Track 4: 'Beledi'

a) Assume starting position.
b) Knees flexed.
c) Feet close together but not touching.
d) Step forward onto the flat of the right foot and, keeping the left foot where it is, raise it slightly up from the floor, then immediately lower it to the floor.
e) Step back onto the flat of the right foot and raise and lower the left foot again.
f) Continue by stepping forward onto the flat of the right foot and raising and lowering the left foot.

Think of it as a rocking motion from one foot to the other. It may help to repeat to yourself as you do it: forward step back step, forward step back step.

Repeat this on the left side:

a) As you step forward onto the flat of the left foot, slightly raise and immediately lower the right foot.
b) As you step back onto the flat of the left foot, slightly raise

and immediately lower the right foot.

Once you have mastered the basic step, include the hip push. Each time you step forward and back on your right foot, push your right hip out. Each time you step forward and back on your left foot, push your left hip out.

Now try the forward-step back-step up on the balls of your feet. Do not drop your heels.

Variation on the forward-step back-step

a) As you step forward onto the ball of your right foot, raise your left leg up behind your right leg just above your ankle. If you are doing it correctly your knee will be bent.

b) As you step back onto the ball of your right foot, raise your left leg up in front of your right foot just above your ankle with the knee bent.

Repeat several times, then change feet:

a) As you step forward onto the ball of your left foot, raise your right leg up behind your left leg just above your right ankle; the knee should be bent.

b) As you step back onto the ball of your left foot, raise your right leg up in front of your left leg just above your right ankle with knee bent.

Forward-step back-step with drop

a) Rise up onto the balls of both feet.

b) Drop forward onto the flat of the right foot.

c) Raise and lower the ball of the left foot.

d) Immediately step back onto the ball of the right foot.

e) You should now be up on the balls of both feet.

f) Drop forward onto the flat of the left foot.

g) Raise and lower the ball of your right foot.

h) Immediately step back onto the ball of the left foot.

i) You should now be up on the balls of both feet.

j) Drop forward onto the flat of the right foot.

k) Raise and lower the ball of your left foot.

Continue the sequence several times.

Change feet:

a) Rise up onto the balls of both feet.

b) Drop forward onto the flat of the left foot.

c) Raise and lower the ball of the right foot.

d) Step back onto the ball of the left foot.

e) Raise and lower the ball of the right foot.

f) Drop forward onto the flat of the left foot.

g) Raise and lower the ball of your right foot.

h) Step back onto the ball of the left foot and continue the sequence.

Double hip twist with forward-step back-step

a) Assume starting position.

b) Stand with feet close together

c) Weight evenly distributed.

d) Knees flexed.

e) Place your right leg forward with heel raised.

f) Twist your right hip inwards twice in quick succession, then step back onto the flat of the right foot.

g) Immediately raise and lower the left foot as in the basic 'step forward step back' step.

h) Bring your right foot through again with the heel raised and twist your hips twice in quick succession again.

i) Step back onto the flat of your right foot and immediately raise and lower your left foot to the floor.

j) Bring your right foot forward and twist the right hip again. Repeat several times, then try the movement on the left.

Dance step pattern

Twist twist back step, twist twist back step

Now try this step turning on the spot.

Step: double hip twist with forward-step back-step pivoting

a) Place your right foot forward with heel raised and do the double hip twist with your right hip.
b) As you step back, transferring your weight onto the flat of your right foot, immediately raise and lower your left foot as you turn a little to the left.
Repeat the movement several times, turning to the left, then change feet and twist your left hip as you turn to the right.

Arms for twist with forward-step back-step

a) Hold your left arm out to the side below shoulder level.
b) Bend your right arm at the elbow so that it is positioned under the rib cage.
c) As you step forward with the right foot, sway your arms over to the right; as you step back with the right foot, sway your arms over to the left.

Hip Twist Walk

Music for hip twist walk
Hossam Ramzy, *Best of Abdul Halim Hafiz*
Side A, Track 1: 'Bahlam Beek'

a) Assume starting position.
b) Stand with your feet close together but not touching.
c) Weight evenly distributed.
d) Rise up onto the balls of both feet.
e) Take small alternate steps forward and practise walking around the room on the balls of your feet.

Now try the walk with the hip twist (don't raise your knees as you twist your hips forward as it makes the step look very awkward and clumsy):

a) As you take a short step forward onto the ball of the right foot, twist your right hip forward.

b) Immediately step forward onto the ball of your left foot and twist your left hip forward.

c) Continue to step and twist your hips alternatively as you travel forward.

This movement is also done with a hip shimmy.

Arm movement

a) Raise your arms out to the side, keeping them below shoulder level.

b) Relax the elbows and raise your hands, with palms facing the floor. Hold the arms steadily in this position as you travel forward. Do not move them to and fro.

Hip Push Travelling

(The Ghawazee dance step)

This movement involves a side-to-side hip push as you travel forward. Because you are travelling forward it is tempting to step forward, but in order to do the movement correctly you must step from side to side; from right to left.

Music for hip pushes

Hossam Ramzy, *Baladi Plus*
Track 3: 'Mashalla'

Solace, *Rhythm of the Dance*
Track 4: 'Beledi'

Assume starting position. Stand with your feet close together; knees flexed.

Practise the walk first:

a) As you step to the right onto the flat of your right foot, immediately raise your left foot slightly off the floor and bring it towards your right foot.

b) As you step to the left onto the flat of the left foot, immediately raise your right foot slightly off the floor and bring it towards your left foot.

c) Repeat, stepping side to side from right to left until you have perfected the basic step.

Now include the hip push by pushing the hip from right to left:

a) As you step to the right, push your right hip out to the right, bring your left foot over to the right.

b) As you step to the left, push your left hip out to the left, bring your right foot over to the left.

Remember, this is done with a side step. Do not step forward; always step out to the side from right to left.

Continue pushing out your hips as you step from side to side on the flat of your feet, then rise up onto the balls of your feet and do exactly the same as you did on the flat of your feet. Eventually you should be able to push your hips from left to right with little effort.

When you are feeling really competent, try the movement travelling backwards, first on the flat of the feet, then up on the balls of the feet.

Travelling double hip pushes

Practise the basic step first, doing two steps to the right:

a) Step to the right onto the flat of your right foot.

b) Bring your left foot up beside your right foot and place it flat on the floor, then step to the right again onto the flat of the right foot, and bring your left foot up beside the right foot.

c) Immediately step to the left onto the flat of the left foot, bring your right foot up beside the left foot and place it flat on the floor.

d) Then immediately step to the left again onto the flat of the left foot, and bring your right foot up beside your left foot. Continue around the room by stepping twice to the right, then twice to the left.

Dance step pattern
Footwork, stepping to the right:
Right foot – left foot – right foot – left foot
Stepping to the left:
Left foot – right foot – left foot – right foot

Now try including the hip pushes:

Dance step pattern
Keeping both feet flat...
a) Step to the right on the flat of the right foot and, as you push your hip to the left, bring your left foot up beside your right foot.
b) Repeat the step again to the right.
c) Then, step to the left on the flat of your left foot and, as you push your hip out to the left, place your right foot beside your left foot.
d) Repeat the step again to the left.

Dance pattern
Count 1 2 3 4 as you...
Step push step push to the right

Count 1 2 3 4 as you...
Step push step push to the left
Once you have mastered the step on the flat of the feet, try it up on the balls of both feet. This step is very effective when done with the hip shimmy.

Arm movement

a) Place your arms down by your side.
b) Raise them up in front of you no higher than bust level, then take them out to the side.
c) Raise the hands.
d) Hold the arms in this position while doing the dance steps.

Travelling Hip Bounces

Music for travelling hip bounces
Chalf Hassan, *Belly Dance from Morocco*
Track 5: 'Solo Darbuka'

This is a lively dance movement that involves using three dance steps simultaneously. When you step back, raise your heel of the foot in front and bounce the hip. Do not move the foot, otherwise you create an extra step.

a) Assume starting position.
b) Stand with your feet close together but not touching.
c) As you step back onto the flat of the right foot, immediately raise your left heel and bounce the left hip twice in quick succession.
d) Step back onto the flat of the left foot, immediately raise your right heel and bounce your right hip twice in quick succession.
Continue the dance step several times.

Variation on travelling hip bounces

a) As you step back onto the flat of your right foot, raise the left heel and do four bounces on your left hip.
b) Step back onto the flat of your left foot, raise your right heel and do four bounces on the right hip.
Continue.

Travelling hip bounces with two bounces forward and two bounces back

a) Assume starting position.

b) Stand with your feet close together but not touching

c) As you step back onto the flat of the right foot, raise your left heel, twist your left hip forward and bounce your left hip twice, then push the left hip back and bounce the hip twice. You should have done four hip bounces on the right side, two forward and two back.

d) Immediately step back onto the flat of the left foot, raise the right heel, twist the right hip forward and bounce your right hip twice, then push the right hip back and bounce the hip twice. You should have done four hip bounces on the right side, two forward and two back.

If you find this movement difficult, just do four hip bounces on the right side and four hip bounces on the left side without the twist. Eventually you will be able to do the two bounces forward and two back.

Variation on hip bounces

Now try doing four hip bounces as you take the hip back and four hip bounces as you take the hip forward:

a) As you step back onto the flat of your right foot, raise your left heel and do four hip bounces back and four hip bounces forward with your left hip.

b) As you step back onto the flat of your left foot, raise your right heel and do four hip bounces back, and four hip bounces forward with your right hip.

Repeat several times.

Arm movement for the travelling hip bounces

a) Raise your arms above your head and relax the elbows.

b) As you step back on your right foot, sway your arms over to the left and hold them in this position until you have done your hip bounces on the left hip.

c) As you step back on your left foot, sway your arms over to the right and hold them in this position until you have done your hip bounces on the right hip.

Steps and bounce with quarter turns

Assume starting position.

Practise the basic step first on the flat of the feet:

a) Step forward onto the flat of your right foot.
b) Step forward onto the flat of your left foot.
c) Do a quarter turn to the right and bounce your left hip twice.

a) Step forward onto the flat of your left foot.
b) Step forward onto the flat of your right foot.
c) Do a quarter turn and bounce your right hip twice.

a) Step forward onto the flat of your left foot.
b) Step forward onto the flat of your right foot.
c) Do a quarter turn to the right and bounce your right hip twice.

a) Step forward onto the flat of your right foot.
b) Step forward onto the flat of your left foot.
c) Do a quarter turn to the right and bounce your left hip.

Dance step pattern

a) Right foot, left foot, turn, then bounce your right hip twice.
b) Left foot, right foot, turn, then bounce your left hip twice.
c) Right foot, left foot, turn, then bounce your right hip twice.
d) Left foot, right foot, turn, then bounce your left hip twice.

If you say it to yourself, you will become familiar with the alternate step pattern:

Forward step, forward step, turn – bounce and bounce

Forward step, forward step, turn – bounce and bounce

When you have mastered the basic step, do it as it should be done – up on the balls of the feet:
a) Step forward onto the ball of the right foot.
b) Step forward onto the ball of the left foot.
c) After you have done a quarter turn lower the right heel.
d) Raise the left heel and bounce the left hip.

a) Step forward onto the ball of the left foot.
b) Step forward onto the ball of the right foot.
c) After you have done a quarter turn, lower the left heel.
d) Raise the right heel and bounce the right hip.
Continue the sequence in quarter turns to the right, then turning to the left.

Travelling Forward Hip Twist

Music for travelling forward hip twist
Burhan Ocal, Istanbul Oriental Ensemble, *Gypsy Rum*
Track 7: 'Nihavent Oyun Havasi'

This is a quick and lively step but do it slowly at first.
a) Assume starting position.
b) Place your right foot directly in front of your left foot.
c) Rise up onto the balls of both feet and practise the walk first without the twist.
d) Step forward on the ball of your right foot, then bring your left foot up behind your right foot, step forward again with the right foot and bring your left foot up behind your right foot.
Repeat the step travelling forward.
a) Change feet, placing the left foot directly in front of your right foot.
b) Rise up onto the balls of both feet.

c) Step forward with the left foot, then bring your right foot up behind your left foot.

Repeat the step travelling forward.

Now try it with the twist, and remember to stay up on the balls of both feet throughout the movement (if you don't, it will look like you're limping):

a) As you step forward with the right foot, twist your right hip inwards.

b) Immediately bring your left foot up behind the heel of your right foot.

c) As you step forward again with your right foot, twist your right hip inwards.

Repeat the step until you have done about twelve, then try it on your left side.

Hip twist travelling to the right and left

When doing these travelling hip twists, you must keep your feet close together, with one foot directly in front of the other and only take a very tiny step. Don't stride out to the side. Do not drop the heels.

a) Rise up onto the balls of both feet.

b) When travelling to the right, place your right leg in front of your left leg. Leading with the right leg, do several hip twists to your right.

c) When you travel to the left, place your left leg in front of your right leg and twist your left hip. Do several hip twists to your left.

Variation on the hip twist

a) Place your right foot in front of your left.

b) Travelling to the right, do sixteen hip twists in a large circle around the floor.

c) Change feet, placing the left foot in front of the right.

d) Travelling to the left, do sixteen hip twists in a large circle around the floor.

e) When you have completed the circle, do eight or sixteen spins to the right on the spot.

a) Place your left foot in front of your right foot.
b) Travelling in a large circle to the left, do sixteen hip twists.
c) When you have completed the circle, do eight or sixteen spins to the left on the spot.

Or: Do eight hip twists completing half a circle and spin to the count of sixteen, then do another eight hip twists to complete the circle and spin to the count of sixteen.

Hip twist with variation

Music for hip twist

Burhan Ocal, Istanbul Oriental Ensemble, *Gypsy Rum*
Track 7: 'Nihavent Oyun Havasi'

Hossam Ramzy, *Eshta*
Track 2: 'Wahda Wahda'
This track starts slowly and builds up to a very quick tempo.

a) Assume starting position.
b) Stand with feet close together, knees flexed.
c) Place your right foot forward and raise the heel. Keep the leg fairly straight, but do not lock the knee.
d) The left foot should be flat on the floor.
e) Do a double twist with your right hip inwards.
f) Keeping the leg forward with the heel raised, take the hip back till your hips are level and bounce your right hip twice.

Dance pattern

Twist~twist bounce~bounce – twist~twist bounce~bounce

Repeat several times. Then try the same movement on the left side.

Pivoting hip twist

Music for hip twists
Hossam Ramzy, *Best of Abdul Halim Hafiz*
Track 2: 'Khusara Khusara'

a) Place your right leg forward with the heel raised, and do a single or double hip twist with your right hip as you pivot to the left.
b) Change feet and place your left foot forward with the heel raised and do a single or double hip twist with your left hip as you pivot to the right.

Pivoting hip twist on the balls of the feet

Music
Hossam Ramzy, *Source of Fire*
Track 6: 'Sahara Groove'

Hossam Ramzy, *Eshta*
Track 2: 'Wahda Wahda'
(starts slowly, then builds up to a quick tempo)

This hip twist is done turning on the spot, up on the balls of the feet, by exchanging weight from one foot to the other as you twist your hip. Think of it as a rocking motion from one foot to the other.

a) Rise up onto the balls of both feet and place your right foot in front of your left foot.
b) Twist your right hip as you turn on the spot to the left.
c) Change feet by placing your left foot in front of your right

foot.

d) Twist your left hip as you turn on the spot to the right.

Arm movement

Use the same arm movements as you used for the other hip pivoting dance steps.

Double hip twists travelling forward

Music

Burhan Ocal, Istanbul Oriental Ensemble, *Gypsy Rum*
Track 7: 'Nihavent Oyun Havasi'

Hossam Ramzy, *Best of Abdul Halim Hafiz*
Track 2: 'Khusara Khusara'

Hossam Ramzy, *Eshta*
Track 2: 'Wahda Wahda'
(starts slowly, then builds up to a quick tempo)

I have to be honest – this is not an easy one to explain in written form. But give it a go by practising the walk first.

Dance step pattern

This is done to a count of "1, 2, 3".

Basic step

a) Assume starting position.
b) Rise up onto the balls of both feet.
c) Step forward on the ball of the right foot, then immediately bring the ball of your left foot up behind the heel of your right foot.
d) Step forward again on the ball of the right foot, then immediately step forward onto the ball of your left foot.

e) Bring the ball of the right foot up behind the heel of your left foot, then step forward again on the ball of the left foot.

f) Immediately step forward onto the ball of your right foot, then bring the ball of your left foot up behind the ball of your right foot.

g) Step forward again onto the ball of your right foot.

h) Step forward again onto the ball of your left foot and continue practising the dance step pattern:

Step right foot, left foot, right foot

Count 1 2 3

Step left foot, right foot, left foot

Count 1 2 3

Now comes the tricky bit when you have to include the double hip twist which   you do as follows:

Each time you step forward and place your weight onto the ball of the right foot, twist your right hip forward. Then do the same as you step forward onto the ball of the left foot. It will help if you say to yourself:

Twist and twist, twist and twist, twist and twist, twist and twist

Don't forget to keep both heels up off the floor throughout the movement. Start slowly at first and, as you perfect the movement, practise it to a quicker tempo.

Arm movement

a) Raise your arms above your head and relax the elbows.

b) As you twist your right hip, sway your arms over to the left; as you twist your left hip sway your arms over to the left.

Basic travelling hip thrust

Music
Hossam Ramzy, *Best of Abdul Halim Hafiz*
Side A, Track 1: 'Bahlam Beek'

Hossam Ramzy, *Best of Mohammed Abdul Wahab*
Track 6: 'Azizi'

Richard Hagopian, Omar Faruk Tekbilek, *Gypsy Fire*
Track 9: 'Beledi'
Track 8: 'Konyali'

a) Assume starting position.
b) Stand with your feet close together, not touching.
c) Knees flexed.
d) Step forward onto the ball of the right foot and, as you do so, push your right hip out and up to the side.
e) Slightly raise the ball of the right foot up off the floor, then step onto the flat of that foot, transferring your weight onto that foot.
f) Now, step forward onto the ball of the left foot and, as you do so, push your left hip up and out to the side.
g) Raise the ball of the left foot slightly off the floor, then step onto the flat of that foot, transferring your weight onto that foot.
h) Step forward onto the ball of the right foot again and, as you do so, push your left hip out and up to the side.
i) Raise the right foot slightly off the floor, then step onto the flat of that foot, transferring your weight onto that foot.
j) Then bring your left foot forward and continue to practise the step.
When stepping forward onto the balls of the feet, do not raise the heel of the other foot.

Dance step pattern

Step push, step push, step push, step push

If you find this movement a little difficult, leave out the hip thrust. Just tap the floor with the ball of your right foot, then step onto the flat of the right foot. Then tap the floor with the ball of your left foot and step onto the flat of the left foot. Once you have got into the rhythm, you will then be able to combine this step with the hip thrust.

Basic travelling hip thrust backwards

a) Assume starting position.
b) Stand with your feet together.
c) Knees flexed.
d) Place your right foot forward with the heel raised.
e) Raise the ball of the right foot slightly up off the floor and, as you lower it to the floor, push your right hip out and up.
f) Immediately step back onto the flat of the right foot.
g) Raise the ball of the left foot slightly off the floor and, as you lower it to the floor, push your left hip out and up, then immediately step back onto the flat of the left foot.
h) Continue the movement by stepping back on alternate feet.

Travelling hip swing

This is not as complicated as it seems. The step is the same as the travelling hip thrust, but instead of pushing your hips out and up alternatively, swing the hip as far forward as you can.

Arm movement for travelling hip swing

a) As you step forward onto the ball of the right foot, place your right arm out to the front just below your bust line with elbow relaxed.
b) Place your left hand at your temple.
c) As you step forward onto the ball of your left foot, extend

your left arm forward.

d) Place your right hand at your temple.

e) As you step forward onto the ball of your left foot, extend your right arm forward and place your left hand at your temple.

The hip push with cross step

This time, instead of stepping forward, you step out to the right, then out to the left side.

a) Assume starting position.

b) Stand with feet close together.

c) Step out to the right side onto the ball of the right foot, and push your right hip out and up. Then...

d) Bring your right foot across the front of your left leg, transferring your weight onto the flat of your right foot.

e) Immediately step out to the left side onto the ball of the left foot, and push your left hip out and up. Then...

f) Bring your left foot across the front of your right foot, transferring the weight onto the flat of your left foot.
Continue to travel forward by stepping out to the right, then crossing your right leg over your left leg, then stepping out to the left and crossing your left leg over your right leg.

Dance step pattern travelling forward

Step to the right, cross with the right
Step to the left, cross with the left

When travelling backwards after stepping out to the right side, place your right foot behind your left leg; then, after stepping out to the left, place your left foot behind your right leg.

Dance step pattern travelling backwards

Step to the right, behind with the right
Step to the left, behind with the left

Arm movements for travelling hip thrusts

a) Raise both arms above your head and relax the elbows.

b) When you step forward onto the right leg, stretch up your right arm, and at the same time bring down your left arm bent at the elbow so it is positioned across the top of your head but not touching your head.

c) As you step forward onto your left foot, stretch up your left arm, and at the same time bring down your right arm bent at the elbow so that it is positioned across the top of your head but not touching your head.

Or, for either dance step:

Sway both arms over to the right as you step forward with your right foot, or place your right foot out to the side. Sway to the left as you step forward with your left foot, or place your right foot out to the side.

Side step with hip push

Music

Hossam Ramzy, *Source of Fire*
Track 6: 'Sahara Groove'

Hossam Ramzy, *Baladi Plus*
Track 3: 'Mashalla'

Assume starting position. Keep your knees flexed. Stand with your feet close together.

When doing this movement both feet must be flat, and the side step and hip push must be done simultaneously.

a) As you step to the right onto the flat of the right foot, push your left hip out to the left. Immediately bring your left foot up to the right foot, then step out to the right again and do another hip push.

b) Repeat several times.

Then try it in the opposite direction.

a) As you step to the left onto the flat of the left foot, push your right hip out to the right. Immediately bring your right foot up to your left foot and step to the right again.
b) Continue to push your right hip out as you step to the left.
c) Now do four hip pushes to the right.
d) Four hip pushes to the left.
e) Two to the right.
f) Two to the left, then repeat the sequence.

Variation on hip push

a) As you step to the right, do one slow hip push with the left hip, followed by two quicker ones.
b) Do several travelling to the right, then as you step to the left do one slow hip push with the hip out to the right, followed by two quicker ones.

Dance pattern

Step to the right and do one slow hip push to the count of 1 2 3 4, followed by the two quicker ones to the count of 1 2, 1 2.

Hip push swing

The hip push swing is done to a quick tempo. Imagine how a pendulum swings from side to side. It is effective when done travelling around in a large circle with your back into the circle so that you are facing your audience.

a) Rise up onto the balls of both feet.
b) As you step to the right, push your right hip out to the right.
c) As you bring your left foot up to your right foot, push your hip to the left.
d) As you step to the right, push your right hip out.
e) As you bring your left foot up to your right foot, push your left hip out.

Hip push swing with drop step

Travel to the right leading with the right foot and right hip. Then travel to the left leading with the left foot and left hip.

a) Rise up onto the balls of your feet and push hips from right to left.

b) Immediately drop onto the flat of both feet and push your hips from right to left.

c) Immediately rise up onto the balls of both feet and push hips from right to left.

d) Immediately drop onto the flat of both feet again and push your hips from right to left.

Dance step pattern

To a count of "1, 2, 3":

1. On the balls of the feet; 2. On the flat of the feet; 3. Up on the balls of the feet

   Push hips right, then left; push hips right, then left; push hips right, then left

Arm movement for side step with hip push

a) Raise your arms above your head and relax the elbows.

b) Sway your arms over to the right, hold them in that position as you travel to the right, then sway your arms over to the left and hold them in that position as you travel to the left.

   Or: When travelling to the right, extend your left arm out to the side below shoulder level, elbow relaxed; right arm across your front, bent at the elbow and held just below bust level.

   When travelling to the left, extend your right arm out to the side; left arm across your front, bent at the elbow.

The Grapevine

Music

Slow to medium tempo as used with side step with hip push.

Assume starting position. Stand with feet close together. Keep the feet flat throughout the movement.

a) Step to the right with the right foot.
b) Bring your left leg across your right leg.
c) Step to the right again with the right foot.
d) Bring your left leg behind the right leg.
e) Step to the right, bring your left leg across your right. Continue travelling to the right.

Dance step pattern

Step to the right, cross with the left, step to the right, behind with your left. Step to the right, across with your left, and continue.

Now try it in the opposite direction.

Step to the left, cross with your right, step to the left, behind with your right. Step to the left, across with your right, continue.

You can also do this dance step on the balls of both feet.

Grapevine with leg elevation

This movement is done on the flat of the feet. Stand with your feet slightly apart and step onto the flat of the feet while doing this movement.

Travelling to the right:

a) Take your right leg behind your left leg.
b) Step to the left on the flat of the left foot.
c) Cross your right leg over your left leg, stepping onto the flat of the foot.
d) Raise your left leg slightly up from the floor, then immediately take your left leg behind your right leg, stepping onto the flat of the left foot.

e) Step to the right onto the flat of the right foot.

f) Cross your left leg over your right leg onto the flat of the left foot.

g) Raise your right leg slightly off the floor.
To repeat, take your right leg behind your left leg.

Grapevine with camel rock

This is done on the flat of both feet.

a) Leading with the right foot, step to the right onto the flat of the right foot.

b) Cross your left leg over your right leg.

c) Step to the right onto the flat of your right foot.

d) Cross your left leg behind your right leg.

e) Rock forward onto the flat of the right foot.

f) Back onto the flat of the left foot.

g) Then forward again onto the flat of the right foot.
Travelling to the left:

a) Leading with the left foot, step to the left onto the flat of the left foot.

b) Cross your right leg over your left leg.

c) Step to the left onto the flat of your left foot.

d) Cross your right leg behind your left leg.

e) Rock forward onto the flat of the left foot.

f) Back onto the flat of the right foot.

g) Then forward onto the flat of the left foot.
Continue by stepping to the right again.

Grapevine with forward-step back-step

Stepping to the right (keep the feet flat):

a) Step to your right onto the flat of your right foot.

b) Cross your left leg over your right leg.

c) Step to the right onto the flat of your right foot.

d) Cross your left leg behind your right leg.

e) Do one or two forward-step back-steps, by stepping

forward onto the flat of the right foot.

Stepping to the left:

a) Cross your right leg over your left.

b) Step to the left onto the flat of your left foot.

c) Cross your right leg behind your left leg.

d) Stepping forward onto the flat of your right foot, do one or two forward-step back-steps.

To continue, step to the right again. The number of forward-step back-steps will depend on the rhythm of the music.

Arms for basic grapevine

Hold them out to the side below shoulder level with elbows relaxed. For the grapevine with camel rock to the right, hold your arms out to the side; then as you do the camel rock, place your right hand on your temple.

When doing the camel rock to the left, place your left hand on your temple.

Arms for the grapevine with the forward-step back-step

Hold your arms out to the side with elbows relaxed. When you do the forward-step back-step with your right foot, sway your right arm across you just under the bust line as you step forward, and out to the side as you step back.

When doing the forward-step back-step to the left, sway your left arm across you just under the bust line, then as you step back take the arm out to the side.

Brush Step

Music for brush step

Various Artists, *Best of Bellydance from Morocco, Egypt, Lebanon, Turkey*

Track 6: Mostafa Sax, 'Fahrah Amira'

The brush step can be done slowly or quickly on the spot, travelling backwards or with a shimmy. When you brush your foot forward you must use the whole of the sole of the foot.

Practise the brush step:

a) Slide (brush) the flat of the right foot forward along the floor until slightly raised from the floor, then place the right foot beside your left foot.

b) Slide (brush) the flat of the left foot forward along the floor until slightly raised from the floor, then place beside your right foot.

Note: Please do not raise your leg too high. Remember, exposing the soles of your feet in certain areas of the Middle East is considered an insult, so always keep your feet close to the floor when you raise them.

Practise the brush step several times, then combine it with the hip movement:

a) Brush your right foot forward, and as you raise the foot slightly up from the floor, lift your right hip, push the hip back, then place your right foot beside your left foot.

b) Brush your left foot forward, and as you raise the foot slightly up from the floor, lift your left hip, push the hip back, then place your left foot beside your right foot.

Now try the movement stepping back:

As you brush your right foot forward, raise and push your hip back, then step back onto the flat of your right foot; then do the same on the left foot.

This step can also be combined with a continuous shimmy once you have mastered the shimmy.

Figure Eights

Music for figure eights

Hossam Ramzy, *Source of Fire*
Track 4: 'Men El Bourkan'

Track 2: 'Manbaa Innar'

Hossam Ramzy, *Best of Mohammed Abdul Wahab*
Track 1: 'Zeina'

And now for something a little gentler. The figure eight is a smooth, graceful and sensual movement of the hips which can be done to a slow or medium tempo. Imagine an outline of a large figure eight on the floor and trace its shape with your hips.

a) Assume starting position.
b) Stand with your feet slightly apart.
c) Flex your knees and hold both your feet firmly to the floor with your weight evenly distributed.
d) Keep your knees as still as possible throughout the movement.
e) Push the right hip forward and out, then push the right hip back.
f) Hold the right hip in that position as you push the left hip forward and out, then push the left hip back.
g) Hold the left hip in that position as you push the right hip forward and out, then push the right hip back.
Repeat the movement several times.

Forward figure eight

This figure eight involves moving the hips in the opposite direction to the previous one.

a) Assume starting position.
b) Stand with your feet apart as wide as your hip line.
c) Flex your knees.
d) As you raise your right heel, twist your right hip forward.
e) Lower your right heel and hold the right hip in that position.
f) Raise your left heel and twist your left hip forward.
g) Lower the left heel and hold the left hip in that position.

h) Raise your right heel and continue.

Repeat several times. Remember to keep your knees flexed when doing the figure eight; bend your knees or move them to and fro.

Vertical figure eight

Here is another version of the figure eight which should be done to a slow to medium tempo.

a) Assume starting position.

b) Stand with your feet apart no wider than your hip line, with knees flexed.

c) Push your right hip out to the right as far as you can.

d) Raise the heel of the right foot, which will lift up your right hip, then bring the hip and heel down at the same time to central position.

You should now be standing with hips level and feet still apart, ready to continue the movement on the left side.

a) Push your left hip out as far as possible, then...

b) Raise the heel of the left foot, which will raise your left hip up. Bring the hip and heel down at the same time to central position.

Repeat several times smoothly and without pausing.

Undulating figure eight

Follow the instructions for the basic figure eight.

a) Do four figure eights as you slowly bend both knees.

b) Do four figure eights as you come up.

Keep the movement smooth. As you bend your knees, don't lean forward – keep your back straight. Repeat several times.

Variation on the undulating figure eight

To help keep your balance, elevate your rib cage, and as you rise up onto the balls of your feet gently pull your tummy in.

Assume starting position.

a) Keeping your feet flat, do four figure eights as you bend your knees.

b) Then, do four figure eights as you rise up onto the balls of your feet.

c) Lower your heels slowly as you begin the four figure eights while bending your knees.

Arms for undulating figure eights
Using your arms will also help your balance.

a) Hold your arms out to the side just below shoulder level, relax elbows.

b) As you rise up onto the balls of your feet, raise your arms until they are above your head, and place your hands back to back or cross them at the wrists.

c) As you lower your heels, bring your arms down to the side just below shoulder level.

Double hip push with figure eight

a) As you push your right hip forward, do two hip pushes in quick succession. Then...

b) Push your right hip back and hold it in this position as you push your left hip forward, do two hip pushes in quick succession.

c) Repeat the figure eight movement several times with the double hip push several times.

Step pattern
Right side, forward push, push, then push back
Left side, forward push, push, then push back

Variation on figure eight
Assume starting position. Feet slightly apart and flat on the floor.

a) Bring the right hip slightly forward and do a double hip

push (push push), then swing the right hip back.

b) Hold the right hip in that position as you push your left hip forward, swing the left hip back, then the right hip forward, and swing back to complete a figure eight.

c) Now do a double push with the left hip, swing the left hip back, then push the right hip forward and back, then the left hip forward and back to complete a figure eight.

Dance pattern

Right hip forward, push~push, swing back hip
Left hip forward, then back
Right hip forward, then back
Left hip forward, push~push

Basic arm movements for figure eights

Raise your arms out to the side keeping them down below shoulder level and relax your elbows.

Oriental arms

This is a lovely, graceful, undulating alternate movement of the arms, perfect with figure eights. But practise it first before combining it with the figure eights.

It's a bit like rubbing your head and patting your tummy at the same time.

a) Hold your arms out to the side just below shoulder level.

b) Raise your right shoulder, then your right elbow, and as you then dip the arm at the elbow raise your hand.

c) As you bring the right arm down, raise your left shoulder, then as you dip the elbow raise your left hand.

Continue the movement by raising the arms alternatively, and when you have perfected it try it with some basic figure eights.

Basic Camel Rock

Music for camel rocks

Hossam Ramzy, *Source of Fire*
Track 2: 'Manbaa Innar'
Track 4: 'Men El Bourkan'

Hossam Ramzy, *Baladi Plus*
Track 4: 'Alla Hai'

The camel rock movement involves a gentle rocking motion of the hips, which is done by shifting the weight from one leg to the other. Have you ever ridden a camel? If so, you should remember how you rocked as the camel walked.

This version is done on the flat of the feet.

Warning: If you have low back pain it is not advisable to do any of the camel rocks as you hyper-extend the back. When your back becomes stronger and pain-free then you can try it, but only gently at first to see how your back copes. If you feel any pain then stop.

Assume starting position. Stand with your feet close together but not touching. Elevate your rib cage and hold this position throughout the movement.

While practising the step, place your hands behind you and rest them gently on the cheeks of your bottom with palms facing outwards (so you don't look like you're grabbing your bottom).

a) As you step forward onto the flat of the right foot, simultaneously contract your abdomen (i.e. pull your tummy in) and stick your bottom out.

b) As you bring your left leg through, relax your abdomen and tilt your pelvis forward and up (a basic pelvic tilt).

c) As you step onto the flat of your left foot, simultaneously contract your abdomen and stick your bottom out.

d) As you bring your right leg through, relax your abdomen

and tilt your pelvis forward and up.

e) Continue by stepping forward again onto the flat of the right foot, then onto the flat of the left foot.

When you have perfected the camel rock, when leading with your right foot step slightly to the right; when leading with the left foot step slightly to the left.

Variation on camel rock 1

This time do a double step on the spot, first to the right, then to the left.

Basic step

a) Step to the right onto the flat of the right foot, transferring your weight onto the right foot.

b) Rock back onto the left foot, transferring your weight onto the left foot then rock forward again, transferring your weight onto the flat of the right foot.

c) Now rock to the left, transferring your weight onto the flat of the left foot.

d) Rock back, transferring your weight onto the flat of the right foot.

e) Rock forward, transferring your weight onto the fat of the left foot.

f) Continue by rocking forward again onto the flat of your right foot.

When you have mastered the basic step, add the rocking motion of the hips; then try this movement travelling forward.

Variation on camel rock 2

Do the same movement you did for the basic camel rock. Instead of travelling forward, turn on the spot to the right, then change feet and turn to the left on the spot.

a) Place your right leg forward and do eight camel rocks,

turning to the right by transferring your weight from your right foot back onto your left foot.

b) Place your left leg forward and do eight camel rocks, turning to the left by transferring your weight from your left foot back onto your right foot.

You can also place your right foot forward and turn to the right. Place your left foot forward and turn to the left.

The camel rock can also be done turning on the spot up on the balls of the feet, with arms raised above your head and hands back to back or crossed at the wrists.

Undulating camel rock

a) Do one camel rock on the flat of the feet.

b) Rise up onto the balls of your feet and do another camel rock.

c) Continue to do another on the flat of the feet, followed by one up on the balls of the feet.

This can be done travelling around to the right, then to the left on the spot.

Or, by facing forward and travelling to the right, then to the left. When doing this version of the camel rock your right foot should stay directly in front of your left foot when travelling to the right, and not out to the side.

Your left foot should stay directly in front of your right foot when travelling to the left, and not out to the side.

Arm movements for camel rocks

Place your arms behind your back and rest the back of the hands gently on the cheeks of your bottom.

Or:

a) As you travel to the right, place your right hand at your temple and your left arm out to the left side below shoulder level with elbow relaxed.

b) When you travel to the left, place your left hand at your temple and hold your right arm to the right with elbow relaxed.

Make sure that when you place your hand at your temple you don't look like you're saluting or pointing one finger at your temple. Use a mirror so that you can see what you are doing.

Or:

a) As you travel to the right, place your right hand at your temple, left hand on your buttock just below the waist with palm facing outwards.

b) When travelling to the left, change the position of your arms so that your left one is placed at your temple, and your right one on your buttock.

Camel rock with hip circle

a) Assume starting position.

b) Place your right foot directly in front of your left foot.

c) Leading with the right foot and travelling to the right, do one camel rock on the flat of the feet.

d) Rise up onto the balls of the feet and do a small hip circle anti-clockwise.

e) Continue to travel to the right, then place your left foot forward.

f) Travelling to the left, do one camel rock on the flat of the feet; then rise up onto the balls of the feet and do one small hip circle clockwise.

Do not step out to the right or left when doing this movement; the feet should stay fairly close together.

Hip Shimmy

Music for hip shimmies

Hossam Ramzy, *Baladi Plus*

Track 5: 'Baladi We Hetta'

Track 7: 'Malfuf Ala Westi'

Chalf Hassan, *Belly Dance from Morocco*
Track 5: 'Solo Darbuka'

Burhan Ocal, Istanbul Oriental Ensemble, *Gypsy Rum*
Track 8: 'Hicazkar Sahin Oyun Havasi'

The shimmy is a very important movement and used widely in the dance combined with a variety of other dance steps. It may take some time to perfect, but do persevere. You cannot do the belly dance without doing a perfect shimmy.

Warning: Numerous teachers, performers and learners use their knees when shimmying their hips. You should not use your knees when doing the shimmy. This action can damage your knees, and has actually damaged the knees of some learners. The hip shimmy should be done from the hips. And it's just as effective if done correctly.

a) Assume starting position.
b) Stand with your feet close together firmly on the floor and weight evenly distributed.
c) Flex knees and hold them as steady as possible.
d) Drop your bottom a little, as though you are about to sit down, but changed your mind.
e) Place your hands firmly together as though in prayer when practising the shimmy. This will stop other parts of your body from moving, particularly your hands, arms and shoulders.
f) To achieve the hip shimmy, shake your hips to a very fast tempo.

Undulating shimmy
a) As you shimmy your hips, bend both knees to a count of four. And rise up to a count of four.
b) Do not lean forward as you bend your knees.
Repeat several times.

Hip shimmy with hip twist

a) As you do the basic hip shimmy, twist your right hip forward to a count of four and then twist your left hip forward to a count of four.
b) Don't stop shimmying.
c) As you continue to shimmy your hips, twist your hips forward and back to a count of "1, 2".
Practise these basic shimmies for as long as you can, then relax.

Travelling hip shimmy

a) Assume the same position as you did for the basic hip shimmy.
b) Lift your feet alternatively as though you are marching on the spot. But do not lift them too high off the floor or raise your knees.
c) Now shimmy your hips.
d) Practise this movement on the spot for several minutes, then travel around the room taking small alternative steps as you shimmy your hips, then...
e) Try the travelling hip shimmy up on the balls of your feet. When you have mastered the basic travelling hip shimmy, try the following.

Hip twist walk with shimmy

Do the basic hip twist as on page 166 and shimmy your hips at the same time. Try it on the flat of the feet, then up on the balls of the feet.

Arabic walk

Practise the walk first, which is a combination of three smooth movements: a lift of the hip, followed by a twist of the hip forward, then a drop of the hip. Take small steps.

a) Rise up onto the balls of both feet.

Belly Dance for Health, Happiness and Empowerment

b) As you step forward onto the ball of the right foot, lift, smoothly twist, then drop the right hip. Then...

c) As you step forward onto the ball of the left foot, smoothly lift, twist, and drop the left hip.

d) Practise this walk until smooth and co-ordinated, then combine it with a continuous hip shimmy.

Hip push shimmy

Music

Hossam Ramzy, *Baladi Plus*
Track 3: 'Mashalla'

Burhan Ocal, Istanbul Oriental Ensemble, *Gypsy Rum*
Track 8: 'Hicazkar Sahin Oyun Havasi'
Plus other tracks of music suitable for shimmies.

a) Assume starting position for shimmy.

b) Stand with your feet apart no wider than your hip line.

c) Flex knees and hold steady.

d) Push your hips out to the right, then out to the left smoothly; when you get into the rhythm do a rapid hip shimmy at the same time.

Variation on the hip push shimmy

a) Assume starting position as with the hip push shimmy.

b) Keep the feet low to the floor and parallel as you lift them alternatively.

c) As you step from right to left, push your hips quickly from right to left and at the same time shimmy your hips in a continuous rapid motion.

When you have got into the rhythm, travel forward and remember to keep your feet parallel as you step from side to side; do not step forward.

Once you have mastered the travelling hip push shimmy on the flat of the feet, try doing it up on the balls of the feet, then travelling backwards. Remember to keep your feet parallel.

Side step with hip push and shimmy
Do the side step as on page 160 with feet flat and combine the step with the hip shimmy.

Continue travelling to the right, then try the movement travelling to the left. Then do the movement up on the balls of the feet.

Arm movements with the shimmies
When doing shimmies keep your arm movements simple.
a) Place your arms down by your side.
b) Bring them forward, keeping the elbows at waist level and relaxed.
c) Take them out to the side, but no wider than hip width, with hands facing down towards the floor or facing upwards towards the ceiling.
d) Hold the arms in this position as you do the shimmies.

Arms with shimmies when travelling to the right or left
a) Raise your arms above your head.
b) Slightly bend your elbows so that your arms are rounded. Then sway your arms over to the left.
c) Hold them in that position as you travel to the right.
d) Sway your arms over to the right and hold them in that position as you travel to the left.

Forward-step back-step with shimmy
Follow the instructions for the basic forward-step back-step on page 156 and as you step forward and back shimmy your hips in a continuous motion.

This step can be done on the flat of the feet, and also up on the balls of the feet.

The forward-step back-step with a shimmy can also be done travelling either to the right or left side. When travelling to the right, lead with your right foot; when travelling to the left, lead with your left foot.

Arm movement for forward-step back-step with shimmy

a) Hold your right arm out to the right, just below shoulder level.

b) Place your left arm across your chest just below your bust.

c) Each time you step forward, smoothly swing both arms over to the right, and every time you step back, swing both arms over to the left.

Hip drop with shimmy

a) Assume starting position as in basic shimmy.

b) Feet close together but not touching.

c) Bend your knees and hold them as steady as you can. Do not move the knees to and fro; this makes the movement jerky and could damage the knees.

d) Drop your hips alternately and at the same time rapidly shimmy your hips.

Side step with hip drop shimmy

Assume starting position. Feet close together, knees flexed and feet flat.

Practise the basic step and take very small steps:

a) As you step to the right onto the flat of the right foot, drop your right hip.

b) As you bring your left foot up beside your right foot, drop the left hip.

c) Immediately step to the right and drop the right hip again.

d) Bring your left foot up to your right foot and drop the left hip again.

Continue travelling to the right.

Change direction and travel to the left:

a) As you step onto the flat of the left foot, drop your left hip.

b) As you bring your right foot up beside your left foot, drop the right hip.

c) Immediately drop your left hip as you step to the left again.

Continue travelling to the left.

Now combine this step with a continuous shimmy.

Dip step with shimmy

Assume starting position. Feet close together but not touching, knees flexed.

Practise the basic step:

a) As you take a small step back onto the flat of the right foot, bend both knees and raise left leg slightly off the floor.

b) Step back onto the flat of the left foot, bend both knees and raise your right leg slightly up from the floor.

c) Now do this movement with a continuous shimmy.

Hip shimmy step

Assume starting position.

a) Rise up onto the balls of both feet and place your right foot directly in front of your left foot.

b) Keeping the feet in this position, take very tiny steps, shimmying your hips as you travel to the right.

c) Place your left foot directly in front of your right foot, and as in (b) shimmy your hips as you travel to the left.

Keep your feet in position as instructed as you travel to the right or left side.

Right and left hip shimmy

Assume starting position.

a) Place your right leg forward with heel raised high.

b) Tighten up the leg muscles from calf to thigh.

c) Now shimmy only your right hip.

d) Change sides and do this on the left hip.

Unless you really tighten those leg muscles, you will find it virtually impossible to do this shimmy.

Left and right hip shimmy

a) Assume starting position.

b) Turn very slightly to the left.

c) Place your right leg out behind you.

d) Raise the right heel.

e) Bend the right knee.

f) Flex the left knee.

g) Shimmy the right hip.

a) Turn very slightly to the right.

b) Place your left leg out behind you.

c) Raise the left heel.

d) Bend the left knee.

e) Flex the right knee.

f) Shimmy the left hip.

Floor shimmy

If you can do this correctly your whole body from your legs upwards will shimmy; it is a very effective movement but difficult to achieve. You would get a better idea of how it should be done if demonstrated by a teacher, but give it a try.

a) Lie on the floor.

b) Make sure your head is aligned with your feet.

c) Place your arms on the floor above your head with hands back to back.

d) Cross your ankles.

e) Raise your bottom up off the floor.

f) Move your ankles up and down very, very quickly.

Shoulder Shimmy

a) Assume the starting position.
b) Stand with your feet slightly apart with knees flexed.
c) Firmly place your hands on the top of your thighs; this will help to keep your shoulders down and relaxed and assist your shoulders to move effortlessly.
d) Move your shoulders to and fro alternatively.
e) Start slowly at first, then gradually quicken the shoulder movement.

Shoulder shimmy with sway

a) Place your hands flat on your thighs.
b) Place your right foot forward on the flat of the foot.
c) Shimmy your shoulders as you sway forward to a count of four, then as you sway back to a count of four.
    When you do this shimmy, do not bend forward and drop your bust. Hold yourself upright as you sway to and fro.

Shoulder shimmy variation

a) Hold your arms up out to the side below shoulder level with elbows relaxed.
b) Stand with feet apart as wide as your hip line and flex your knees.
c) Shimmy your shoulders as you sway over to the right, then immediately sway over to the left while shimmying your shoulders.

When you can do the shoulder shimmy on the spot, swaying forward and back, and travelling forward or backwards effortlessly, raise your arms up a little in front of you, take them out to the side, and hold them steady. Don't hold them too high as this will prevent you from shimmying your shoulders effectively.

Now practise the shoulder shimmy walking around the room on the flat of the feet, then up on the balls of the feet. It's difficult at first not to shimmy your hips at the same time, but if you isolate correctly this will help.

Now combine the shoulder shimmy with the hip shimmy as you walk around the room on the flat of the feet, then up on the balls of the feet.

Shoulder movement

Assume starting position. Raise your arms slightly out to the sides with elbows slightly dipped at waist level; do not pull your shoulders back.

a) Push your right shoulder forward, and as you pull your right shoulder back, push your left shoulder forward.

b) Continue to push your shoulders to and fro alternatively. Do not shimmy your shoulders.

Shoulder roll

Assume starting position.

Holding your arms in the same position:

a) Raise your right shoulder and roll it back; hold it in that position as you raise your left shoulder and roll it back.

b) Hold your left shoulder in that position as you roll your right shoulder back.

Continue raising and rolling your shoulders back alternatively.

Shoulder movement: combination 1

a) Slowly roll your right shoulder back.

b) Slowly roll your left shoulder back.

c) Then do four alternative shoulders rolls in quick succession.

Repeat several times.

Count for slow shoulder roll: 1 2, 1 2

Count for the quicker shoulder roll: 1 2 3 4, 1 2 3 4

Shoulder movement: combination 2

a) Roll your shoulders back alternatively four times.
b) Right shoulder, left shoulder, right shoulder, left shoulder.
c) Raise your right shoulder, then bring it forward and drop it down.
d) Raise your left shoulder, then bring it forward and drop it down.

Repeat the combination several times.

Shoulder movement: combination 3

Place your right foot forward and do any of these shoulder combinations, swaying forward and back:

a) Bring your right shoulder forward to a count of 1, then bring your left shoulder forward to a count of 1.
b) Then bring your shoulders forward alternatively to a count of 4, i.e.

1 2 3 4

Right left right left

Repeat several times.

Shoulder movement: combination 4

This takes a little more concentration, so do it slowly at first.

Arms

a) Assume starting position.
b) Stand with feet close together but not touching, knees flexed.
c) Hold arms down by your side.
d) Raise them up out to the side so that the elbows are level with your waist and slightly dip the elbows. Hold the arms steady in that position throughout the movement.

a) Stand facing the front, then...
b) Turn your body at an angle to the left so that you are facing

a corner.

c) Raise your right shoulder, bring it forward and drop it.

d) Hold it in that position.

e) Raise your right heel, raise your right hip, then twist it forward and drop it, and hold in that position.

f) Pivot slightly to the right so that your body is at an angle and you are facing the opposite corner. Immediately shimmy your shoulders to a count of four. Then...

a) Raise your left shoulder.

b) Drop your left shoulder forward and hold in that position.

c) Raise your heel and left hip.

d) Twist your left hip forward, drop it and hold in that position.

e) Pivot slightly to the left so that your body is at an angle and you are facing the opposite corner.

f) Immediately shimmy your shoulders to a count of four. Repeat the sequence several times.

Shoulder and hip combination

a) Face forward.

b) Stand with feet close together but not touching.

c) Raise your right heel.

d) Raise and drop your right shoulder forward and hold it in that position.

e) Raise and drop your right hip forward.

f) Step to the right onto the flat of the right foot, bring your left foot up to the right foot with heel raised.

g) Shimmy your shoulders to a count of four.

a) Raise and drop your left shoulder forward.

b) Raise and drop your left hip forward.

c) Step to the left onto the flat of the left foot, bring your right foot over to the left foot with heel raised.

d) Shimmy your shoulders to a count of four.

Spins and Turns

Music for spins and turns
Hossam Ramzy, *Best of Mohammed Abdul Wahab*
Track 2: 'Set Elhabayib Ya Habiba'
Track 4: 'Ollo Amallak Eih Albi'

If you have never done spins before, please be very careful as you may experience some dizziness, become disorientated and lose your balance. If you find them difficult, or are not used to spinning, for safety reasons do not attempt to do them, especially when you are alone.

Spinning is a movement that is generally taught in ballet dance classes at a young age and is a difficult movement to achieve as you get older. If you are persistent and have good balance it is possible to learn to spin without getting dizzy.

For those of you determined to master spins, try the following exercises:

a) When spinning to the right, keep your right foot flat on the floor and raise your left heel.

b) Hold your right arm out in front of you at shoulder level, and hold the hand up.

c) Focus on your hand as you start to spin slowly to the right.

d) Gradually increase the speed of your spin, still focusing on your hand. It is said that if you continue to spin in this manner, you will eventually spin yourself out of dizziness, but I don't encourage it unless you're with someone who is a trained dancer and can advise you.

If you feel confident, try this spin in the opposite direction by placing your left arm forward and focusing on your left hand.

There is another way of preventing dizziness when turning or spinning – by focusing on an object directly in front of you, and turning your head round at a precise moment. However, this is a difficult movement to master and one that should be taught and demonstrated by a trained dancer who can do it with ease.

Spins with the hip shimmy

This is a very effective dance movement, but will take some considerable practice. As you spin, shimmy your hips at the same time. It can be done, so keep practising.

If you can spin effortlessly, try the following:
a) Bend over to the right as you spin to the right.
b) Bend over to the left as you spin to the left.

Arm movement with spins

a) When you spin to the right, raise your right arm above your head and bend it at the elbow so that you have a nice curve of the arm.

b) Hold your left arm down by your side and push out the elbow until you have a gentle curve of the left arm, then push the arm back a little.

When you spin to the left, smoothly change the position of your arms. You may prefer to hold both arms out to the side, below shoulder level with elbows relaxed as you spin. But be careful not to drop or raise the arms.

Arms for turns and spins

Practise these arm movements before combining them with the turn:

a) Hold both arms up in front of you below shoulder level and rounded at the elbows. Hands should not touch.

b) Take both arms out to the side, keeping them below shoulder level.

c) Bring them forward again, rounding them at the elbow, and keep the hands apart.

d) Take both arms out to the side again.

Repeat several times, then combine the arm movement with the turn, or spin.

As instructed in arms for turns:

a) Hold your arms out in front of you as instructed.

b) As you step to the right, take your arms out to the side.

c) As you commence your turn to the right, bring your arms forward and keep your hands apart.

d) As you step out to the right side, again take your arms out. Repeat two or three times to the right with the arms in position, then change arms and turn or spin in the opposite direction.

Upper Torso Circle and Combinations

Music
Hossam Ramzy, *Best of Abdul Halim Hafiz*
Side B, Track 1: 'Ganalhawa'

Some of the following movements can be rather exhausting and also cause a little disorientation or dizziness. These movements are not advisable if you have a neck problem. Only practise one or two at a time. If you do suffer from any of these effects then do not do these movements. You need to be fit and supple to try these movements.

a) Assume starting position.

b) Stand with feet apart at hip width, knees flexed.

c) Bend to the right as far as you can.

d) Swing your upper torso forward, down, then over to the left and up.

e) Arch back as far as you can, then repeat the movement two or three times.

Upper torso circle with hip circle

Music

Hossam Ramzy, *Best of Abdul Halim Hafiz*
Side B, Track 1: 'Ganalhawa'

a) Assume starting position.
b) Stand with your feet as wide as your hip line.
c) Knees flexed.
d) Push your left hip out to the left.
e) Bend your upper torso to the right.
f) As you swing your upper torso forward and down, push your hips back.
g) As you swing your upper torso over to the left, push your hips over to the right.
h) Swing your hips forward and over to the left as you bring your upper torso up.

Do several movements to the right and then to the left.

To start the movement to the left, push your right hip out to the right and bend your upper torso to the left.

Double upper torso circle

This movement is based on the same principle as the basic upper torso circle. Bend over to the right again and continue to do another one or two more upper torso circles from right to left.

Try it in the opposite direction by bending over to the left and swinging your upper torso over to the right and continue to do another one or two upper torso circles swinging from left to right.

If you are really flexible and have long hair you should be able to brush the floor with your hair as you swing your upper torso in a circular motion. It can look very effective.

This time, do one large upper torso circle followed by two smaller and quicker ones.

a) Assume starting position.

b) Stand with your feet at hip width, flex knees.

c) Bend your upper torso to the right.

d) Swing forward, over to the left and up.

e) Immediately do two upper torso circles in very quick succession in the same direction.
Relax, then try again. Then practise the same movement in the opposite direction.

Circle with upper torso drop

Assume starting position. Stand with feet apart and knees flexed.

a) Do one large hip circle, then...

b) Bend forward quickly until your head almost touches the floor, and immediately rise up till you are upright.
This is another movement that looks most effective if you have long hair.

Arms for circle with upper torso drop

a) Hold arms out to the side with elbows at waist level; as you drop your upper torso, swing arms gently back.

b) As you raise your torso, bring your arms out to the side again with elbows relaxed.

Upper torso drop with hip circle

a) Bend forward until your head almost touches the floor, immediately rise up, then...

b) Place your right leg forward with heel raised and circle your right hip anti-clockwise.

c) Drop forward, rise up, then place your left foot forward with heel raised and circle your left hip clockwise.
Usually when doing a routine you would only do this once, i.e. not do the movement on the right side then repeat on the left side.

Arms for torso drop with hip circle

a) Hold your arms out to the side with elbows relaxed.
b) As you drop your torso forward, gently swing your arms back.
c) Raise yourself up, then...
d) Simultaneously place your right foot forward and raise your left arm up above your head, curved at the elbow.
e) Place your right arm down by your side, curved to frame your right hip as you circle your right hip anti-clockwise.

Circle within a Circle Combinations

Music

Hossam Ramzy, *Best of Abdul Halim Hafiz*
Side B, Track 1: 'Ganalhawa'

Now we are going back to the basic circle within a circle from page 141. This circle within a circle includes a combination of one large hip circle immediately followed by two smaller circles. It is not an easy movement to achieve and is one that frustrates many of my learners. But it is worth persevering with as it is a lovely movement once mastered.

Practise the basic step first before combining it with the hip circle.

a) Assume starting position.
b) Stand with feet apart, no wider than hip width and parallel.
c) Knees flexed.
d) To complete a half turn, raise your right foot slightly off the floor.
e) Gently swing your right leg forward and step onto the flat of the right foot.
f) You should have completed the half turn and be facing in the opposite direction.

g) Feet should still be apart and parallel.

h) Take two smaller steps forward onto the flat of your right foot as you pivot on the flat of your left foot to the left. You should now be facing your starting position again.

Now try combining those steps with the hip circles:

a) Simultaneously stick your bottom out, swing your right leg forward, and circle your hips anti-clockwise (from right to left).

You should have completed a half turn, finishing with both feet flat and parallel.

b) Now do two smaller hip circles in the same direction to bring you back to your starting position.

Do several of these movements to the right, then repeat in the opposite direction, by sticking your bottom out as you swing your left foot forward and circle your hips clockwise (from left to right) to complete a half turn, then do two smaller hip circles to bring you back to the starting position.

Single pivoting hip circle

Instead of doing three hip rotations, one large and two small, you are going to do just one large pivoting hip circle. You will need good co-ordination, balance and perseverance to perfect this movement, but it can be done.

Practise the turn first without the hip circle. Don't raise the leg up too high or you will lose your balance. Keep it close to the floor.

a) Assume starting position.

b) Feet apart no wider than hip width and parallel.

c) Knees flexed.

d) To complete a full turn to the left, raise your right leg slightly off the floor, swing the leg as far forward as you can as you pivot to the left, before stepping onto the flat of the right foot.

If you have done this correctly, you should now be back where you started from.

Practise this basic step several times to the left and right, then combine it with one large hip circle. This is not an easy movement to explain on paper, but I hope you will get the gist of it.

To complete a smooth large hip circle anti-clockwise (from right to left):
a) Simultaneously, stick your bottom out as you swing your right leg forward as far as you can, and do a complete circle of your hips as you pivot to the left on the flat of the left foot.
b) As you step onto the flat of the right foot, you should now be back at your starting position, having completed the hip circle in one move, and standing with feet apart and parallel.

Relax, repeat two or three times, then try it in the opposite direction. This is when I usually get a moan, in good humour, from the learners as they tend to find moving from left to right a little more difficult.
a) Simultaneously stick your bottom out as you swing your left leg forward as far as you can, and do a complete circle of your hips clockwise (from left to right) as you pivot on the flat of the right foot to the right.
b) As you step onto the flat of the left foot you should be back at your starting position, having completed the circle in one move, and standing with feet apart and parallel.

Pivoting double hip twist with hip rotation
Assume starting position.
a) Feet close together, knees flexed.
b) Place your right leg forward and raise the heel.
c) Depending on the rhythm of the music, do two or three double hip twists as you pivot to the left on the flat of the

left foot.

d) Place the right foot flat on the floor and immediately follow the twists with a hip circle from right to left (anti-clockwise) which should bring you around to face the front.

Do several turning to the left, then change feet and repeat the movement turning to the right, circling your hips clockwise (from left to right):

a) Place your left leg forward with heel raised.
b) Do two or three double hip twists as you pivot to the right on the flat of the right foot.
c) Immediately follow the twists with a circle of your hips from left to right (clockwise).

This combination can be done with hip drops, twists or hip pushes.

Hip circle with pelvic tilt

Music
Hossam Ramzy, *Best of Abdul Halim Hafiz*
Side B, Track 1: 'Ganalhawa'

a) Assume starting position.
b) Stand with feet close together and knees flexed.
c) Place your right leg forward, raise the heel and bend the knee.
d) Circle your right hip slowly once, anti-clockwise, then do a pelvic tilt.
e) Do several on your right side, then try it on your left side.

Hip circle with pelvic tilt and hip drops
a) Assume starting position.
b) Stand with your feet close together but not touching and flex knees.

c) Place your right leg forward, raise the heel and bend the knee.

d) Circle your right hip slowly once, anti-clockwise.

e) Follow the circle with one pelvic tilt, two hip drops back and two hip drops forward.

Repeat several times on the right side, then do the same movement on the left side several times.

Pivoting hip combinations

These pivoting movements can be done with hip bounces or hip pushes.

Assume starting position.

a) Stand with feet close together but not touching.

b) Raise right heel.

c) Do two double hip bounces as you pivot to the left, then...

d) Do three single bounces on the spot.

Continue until you have perfected the movement, then change feet and try it in the opposite direction.

Dance step pattern

Bounce~bounce – bounce~bounce – bounce~bounce~bounce

Count 1 2 – 1 2 – 1 2 3

Depending on the rhythm of the music, you may have to do two double hip bounces followed by four single bounces.

Pivoting hip bounce forward and backwards

a) Facing the front, do four double bounces pivoting to the left. You should now be facing in the opposite direction.

b) Keeping the transition smooth, lower the heel of your right foot, immediately raise the heel of your left foot, then do four double bounces as you push yourself backwards. You should now be facing the front again.

Variation on hip bounce

a) Assume starting position.
b) Stand with feet close together. Raise the right heel.
c) Bounce your right hip twice: bounce, bounce.
d) Push your right hip back and do one bounce.
e) Twist the right hip forward and do one bounce.

Dance step pattern
Bounce~bounce, back and bounce, forward and bounce

Hip drop and bounce combination

a) Push the right hip back and drop the hip once.
b) Twist the hip forward and drop the hip once.
c) Push the hip back and do two quick bounces.
d) Then one forward drop.

Dance step pattern
Back drop, forward drop, back bounce~bounce, forward drop
Try these combinations on the left side.

Travelling hip twists with forward-step back-steps
When travelling to the right, keep your left foot immediately behind your right foot. When travelling to the left, keep your right foot immediately behind your left foot.

a) Assume starting position.
b) Feet close together, knees flexed.
c) Place your right foot forward and raise both your heels.
d) Leading with your right leg, do four hip twists travelling to the right, followed by two forward-step back-steps on your left foot. Then...
e) Leading with your left leg, do four hip twists travelling to the left and two forward-step back-steps on your right foot.

You should now be ready to travel to the right again. Repeat this combination several times.

Hip twists followed with a spin

a) Assume starting position.
b) Stand with your feet close together.
c) Place your right foot forward and rise onto the balls of both feet.
d) Travel to the right, leading with your right foot, and do sixteen hip twists in a large circle around the room.
e) When you have done sixteen hip twists you should be back to your starting position facing the front.
f) Keeping the transition smooth, spin to the right to eight counts.

If you're feeling energetic, spin to sixteen counts. Or: spin to the right for eight counts, then to the left for eight counts.

Leading with the left foot, repeat the combination to the left and do sixteen hip twists, finishing with the spins.

Shimmy with hip pushes

Music

Chalf Hassan, *Belly Dance from Morocco*
Track 4: 'Shela'

a) Assume the starting position.
b) Stand with both feet flat and slightly apart and keep them parallel throughout the movement.
c) Knees flexed.
d) Shimmy your hips to a count of four, then do a double hip push to the right and a double hip push to the left.

Step pattern

Say to yourself as you do it:

Shimmy, shimmy, shimmy, shimmy, right hip, push~push, left hip, push~push

Shimmy, shimmy, shimmy, shimmy, right hip, push~push, left hip, push~push

Repeat several times, then relax.

Now try the same movement with a half turn:

a) Shimmy to a count of four, then do a double push to the right, and a double hip push to the left.

b) As soon as you have done your last hip push, turn to the left, so that you are facing in the opposite direction.

c) Repeat the sequence, then turn to the left; you should now be facing the front again.

Repeat the sequence several times.

Step pattern

Shimmy~shimmy, shimmy~shimmy, push~push, push~push
– turn

Shimmy~shimmy, shimmy~shimmy, push~push, push~push
– turn

Count 1 2 3 4 1 2 1 2

Shimmy and hip circles

a) Stand with feet close together but not touching.

b) Do two small hip circles (anti-clockwise), then shimmy to a count of four.

c) Do two small hip circles in the opposite direction (clockwise), then shimmy to a count of four.

Step Turns

Music for turns and spins

Hossam Ramzy, *Best of Mohammed Abdul Wahab*

Track 2: 'Set Elhabayib Ya Habiba'

Turns
a) Assume starting position.
b) Stand with feet close together, knees flexed.
c) Step to the right onto the flat of the right foot.
d) Swing your left leg forward until you are facing in the opposite direction.
e) Swing your right leg back; you should now be facing the front again.

You should have done three half turns to the right.

Now try the turns to the left:

a) Step to the left onto the flat of the left foot.
b) Swing your right leg forward until you are facing in the opposite direction.
c) Swing your left leg back; you should now be facing the front again.

Step turn with hip drop
a) After you have completed your step turn to the right, raise your left heel and do a hip drop on your left hip.
b) After you have completed your step turn to the left, raise your right heel and do a hip drop on your right hip.

Step: variations with step turn
a) After completing a step turn to the right, instead of doing a hip drop do a quick pelvic tilt.
b) Complete a step turn to the left and do a quick pelvic tilt.
   Now complete a step turn to the right, do a pelvic tilt, and after your step turn to the left do a very quick rib-cage lift.

Step: travelling hip thrusts with turn
a) Starting on the right foot, do three travelling hip thrusts forward, then immediately turn/spin on the spot to the

right.

After completing the turn/spin you should be facing forward.

b) Starting on your left foot, do three travelling hip thrusts forward, immediately followed by a turn/spin on the spot to the left.

Pivoting hip thrust with turn/spin

Assume starting position.

a) Place right leg forward with heel raised and do three double pivoting hip thrusts, turning to the left.

b) Immediately come up onto the balls of both feet and turn/spin on the spot to the left to face the front.
Lower both heels.

a) Place your left leg forward with heel raised and do three double pivoting hip pushes, turning to the right.

b) Immediately come up onto the balls of both feet and turn/spin on the spot to the right to face the front.
Lower both heels.

a) Place your right leg forward and do three double hip pushes, then turn.

b) Repeat six times.

Travelling hip twist with spin/turn

Assume starting position. Feet close together but not touching, knees flexed.

a) Rise up onto the balls of both feet.

b) Place your right leg forward and do four or eight hip twists travelling forward.

c) Step to the left onto the flat of the left foot and do two spins or turns to the left.

d) Place your left foot forward and do four or eight hip twists travelling forward.

e) Step to the right onto the flat of the right foot and do two spins or turns to the right.

To vary this movement, do the Arabic walk (see page 191) with turns/spins.

Rib Cage and Tummy Movements

Music for rib cage and tummy movements

Various Artists, *Beginner's Guide to Bellydance: CD1 Traditional & Cabaret*

Track 1: Phil Thornton, Hossam Ramzy, 'On the Transit of Venus' (New World Music Ltd)

Hossam Ramzy, *Best of Mohammed Abdul Wahab*
Track 3: 'Khai Khai'

Solace, *Rhythm of the Dance*
Track 1: 'Beledi'

Some rib cage movements can cause a little discomfort in the lower back, especially if you have a low back problem, so only do three or four movements at a time until your lower back has strengthened. If any of the rib cage movements cause pain or discomfort in either the lower or upper back then please do not do them.

Rib cage slide

If you isolate correctly, it will enable you to move your rib cage effortlessly while keeping the hips still. Keep your rib cage elevated and shoulders down throughout the movements. Only your rib cage should move.

a) Assume starting position.
b) Stand with your feet slightly apart, knees flexed.
c) Place your hands on your hips or hold them out to the side.
d) Tighten the cheeks of your bottom.

e) Slide your rib cage over to the right, then slide your rib cage over to the left.

Repeat several times, then relax.

Travelling rib cage slides

This one you will really have to think about.

a) Elevate your rib cage.
b) Stand with your feet close together, knees flexed
c) As you take a small step forward onto the flat of your right foot, slide your rib cage over to the right, then over to the left. Then...
d) As you take a small step forward onto the flat of the left foot, push your rib cage back over to the right, then over to the left.

If you slide your rib cage over to the right as you step onto the right foot, then over to the left as you step onto the left foot, you will look a little bit like a pigeon. So follow the instructions carefully.

Practise the rib cage walk for 2–3 minutes, then relax.

Rib cage lifts

a) Elevate rib cage.
b) Stand with feet close together but not touching, knees flexed.
c) Place hands firmly on your hips.
d) Pushing forward from your diaphragm, lift your rib cage, then lower it.

Do not pull your shoulders back as you raise your rib cage as it will make the movement ineffective.

Repeat several times, then relax.

Rib cage pushes

a) Assume the same position as you did for the rib cage slide and lift.

b) This time push the rib cage forward, then pull back.

c) Do not pull your shoulders back as you push your rib cage forward.

Repeat several times, then relax.

Both the rib cage push and rib cage lift can be done travelling forward. With each step you take, raise and lower the rib cage. The same applies to the rib cage push; with each step, push then pull back the rib cage.

Rib cage rolls

The rib cage roll is a combination of the rib cage lift and rib cage push and should be a sensuous and snake-like movement. You need a fairly strong back to do this one, so be careful. If you have low back problems this movement is not advisable. Even if you're fit don't do any more than four at a time.

a) Assume the starting position with rib cage well elevated.

b) Feet slightly apart, knees flexed.

c) Place your hands firmly on your hips while practising.

d) Push your rib cage forward.

e) Lift your rib cage.

f) Pull back the rib cage and push down.

g) Immediately push forward again.

You should have now completed a rib cage roll. Repeat the movement three or four times, then relax.

Travelling rib cage rolls

When you have mastered the rib cage roll on the spot, try the rib cage roll travelling forward. As you step forward onto the flat of the right foot, complete a rib cage roll, then step forward onto the flat of the left foot and complete another rib cage roll.

Repeat three or four times, then relax.

Rib cage circles

This movement can be quite a difficult one to master, therefore it is very important to isolate correctly. Remember that isolation means not moving the lower part of your body as you move your top half, or vice versa.

a) Assume starting position.

b) Feet slightly apart, knees flexed.

c) Elevate your rib cage, and hold the cheeks of your bottom in as tightly as you can.

d) If you place your hands on your hips firmly it should help you to keep your hips from moving until you have mastered the art of isolation.

e) Slide your rib cage over to the right.

f) From this position, push the rib cage forward.

g) Slide over to the left and from this position, pull your rib cage back, and then roll it over to the right.

You should now have completed a full circular movement of the rib cage; repeat the rib cage circle by pushing forward again.

Now this is where the fun begins – trying the rib cage circle in the opposite direction, and believe me, it is not easy, as the majority when dancing or exercising favour the right side, but do persevere.

a) Slide your rib cage over to the left.

b) Push forward from the left, then slide over to the right.

c) From that position, pull the rib cage back and roll it over to the left.

d) Push forward from the left to complete another circle.

e) Do as many as you can to the left, then relax.

Rib cage figure eight

a) Assume the starting position.

b) As in the other rib cage movements you must keep your rib cage elevated throughout the movement.

c) Stand with your feet slightly apart, knees flexed.

d) Place your hands firmly on your hips to prevent them

moving.

e) Slide your rib cage to the right.

f) Push forward from that position and slide the rib cage over to the centre, i.e. over to its natural position.

g) Pull the rib cage back, then slide the rib cage over to the left.

h) Push the rib cage forward, then slide the rib cage back to central position.

i) Pull the rib cage back and repeat the movement from (e) to (i).

All rib cage movements should be smooth, so keep practising to perfect.

Rib cage roll arching back

This is a graceful movement, but it can cause a little strain on the back if you are not very supple. Only try this movement once or twice to begin with. If it does strain your back then please do not attempt to do any more until your back has strengthened.

a) Stand with your feet close together, place the right foot slightly forward and raise the heel.

b) Elevate your rib cage.

c) Push your rib cage out (i.e. forward).

d) Raise your rib cage as in the rib cage lift.

e) Then as you begin to arch back, pull back and push down the rib cage, then stretch forward and repeat the movement.

Arms

You can just frame your hips with your arms or try the following arm movement:

a) Extend your arms out to the side so that your elbows are at waist level.

b) As you push your rib cage forward, raise your arms up above your head.

c) As you pull your rib cage back and down as you arch your back, cross your arms and slowly bring them down in front of you then out and up to the sides, ready to repeat the movement.

Back bend

Not every dancer or learner is supple or flexible enough to do a back bend from a standing position, so please do not attempt this movement if your back is stiff or you have a back problem. When doing a back bend never keep your head up as you could hurt your neck and strain your shoulders. Your head should follow the line of your body.

a) Stand with your feet no wider than hip width.

b) Arch back as far as you can.

c) Hold this position for a few seconds, then slowly come up. If you are proficient at doing the back bend, stand with your feet close together and raise your right heel. While keeping the heel raised, arch back as far as you can, then slowly come up.

Brush step with rib cage roll

This movement should be done smoothly and gently. Instructions for the brush step are on page 181. Instructions for the rib cage roll are on page 218.

a) Assume starting position.

b) Stand with feet close together but not touching.

c) Both the brush step and rib cage roll should be done simultaneously.

d) As you brush your right foot forward, do a rib cage roll.

e) As you brush your left foot forward, do another rib cage roll.

Repeat several times on alternate sides.

Rib cage slide and hip push

a) Assume starting position.
b) Stand with feet apart as wide as your hip line.
c) Flex knees slightly more than you normally would.
d) Hold your arms out to the side just below shoulder level and relax elbows.
e) As you slide your rib cage over to the right, gently push your hips over to the left as far as you can, then...
f) As you slide your rib cage over to the left, push your hips gently over to the right as far as you can.
Be careful not to bend over to the right or left when doing this movement; hold your upper torso up straight. Repeat several times.

Abdominal Rolls and Flutters

Music for abdominal rolls and flutters
Hossam Ramzy, *Best of Mohammed Abdul Wahab*
Track 1: 'Zeina'

Tummy flutter

a) Assume starting position. Rib cage must be elevated.
b) Stand with feet slightly apart, knees flexed.
c) Push your tummy in and out as quickly as you can. With practice you should be able to flutter your tummy with ease. You can do this in two ways, by breathing gently and normally, or by inhaling and holding your breath. So try it both ways to see which gives you the most effective tummy flutter.
d) Keep fluttering for as long as you can, then relax and try again.
Now choose a rhythmic piece of music and pull your tummy in and out in time to the beat of the music.

Pattern

For example, 'out out' is two tummy pushes and 'in in' means pull your tummy in twice. Now follow this sequence:

in out – in out – in out – in out – in out –
in in – out out – in out – in in – out in – out in – out out – in
out – in out

Abdominal roll

Assume starting position. Stand with your feet slightly apart, knees flexed.

To help you get the feel of the tummy roll, practise it with the following deep breathing method.

Warning: Do not attempt this method more than four times, for if you are not used to using the diaphragm when deep breathing, you may hyperventilate, i.e. feel a little dizzy or light-headed. However, if you practise the breathing exercises on pages 61–63 this problem will definitely improve.

a) Exhale and push your tummy out, just let it flop.
b) As you inhale slowly, pull your tummy in – imagine you are trying to touch your spine with it; now pull your tummy up (you should have a hollow under your rib cage) and hold for a second. Then…
c) Exhale slowly through your nose as you push your tummy out and down.

You should have completed a tummy roll. Relax, then try a few more.

Once you have mastered the tummy roll with the deep breathing method, try it breathing as you would normally breathe.

Rib cage roll and tummy roll: combination 1

Assume starting position.

a) One rib cage roll.
b) One abdominal roll.

c) Then do several tummy flutters.

d) Repeat several times until you can do the combination smoothly.

Rib cage roll and tummy roll: combination 2

a) One rib cage roll.

b) Two figure eights.

c) Place right leg forward and do a hip circle anti-clockwise, followed by one camel rock to the right.

d) Do another rib cage roll.

e) Two figure eights.

f) Place your left leg forward and do a hip circle clockwise.

g) Then one camel rock to the left.

(Sources: Tina Hobin, *Belly Dance for Health and Relaxation*, Duckworth Publishers; Tina Hobin, *Belly Dance: The Dance of Mother Earth*, Marion Boyars Publishers)

Choreography

The choreography process is exhausting. It happens on one's feet after hours of work, and the energy required is roughly equivalent of writing a novel and winning a tennis match simultaneously.
(Agnes de Mille, *Dance to the Piper*, 1952)

Definition of choreography: the art of arranging dance steps and movement. The role of a choreographer is to create the art and technique of dance steps, dance patterns and movement; to express and explore new ideas in different disciplines, and understand the creative process.

Choreography is a specialised skill and art form and because one is a dancer it doesn't mean you can be a successful choreographer. To come up with fresh ideas, create something original, is one of the most difficult things to do. Even professional choreographers have days when inspiration and creativity eludes them.

Choreography is a complex art and there is much to learn to become an accomplished choreographer. It is not a question of just putting some movements together and presenting it on stage. You have to have an understanding of the concept of choreography: the theoretical, practical and visual, and understand the concept of space and levels and how one perceives space and levels. A skilled choreographer should be spontaneous, positive and constructive, have a great deal of patience and be a good leader. Not all your dancers will be able to execute your artistic interpretation or be capable of reaching the standards you require so, however frustrating it is, you will have to adapt.

Do not slavishly follow someone else's ideas or compositions, step by step, as such performances lack feeling and artistic interpretation. Although you can gain immense inspiration from the work of others, originality is very important. You need to be innovative and able to think of new ideas, clear your mind and explore your inner source, discover something for yourself. So improvise and see what develops.

1. Be fully committed to the project; you'll never succeed with a half-hearted approach.
2. Think about what you are going to do and how you are going to present it.
3. Music is important so choose carefully. The rhythm and tempo of the music will determine the organisation of dance steps, pattern, movement and mood.
4. Outline your dance and the structure of the dance.
5. Visualise your piece of choreography.
6. Communicate with your dancers and explain what you are doing.
7. When you first start, try not to be too ambitious.
8. Keep the routine short; this will leave your audience wishing for more.
9. Take a look at the size of stage or floor space, and the number of dancers it will accommodate. If that is not possible, contact the organisers and get the details from them, i.e. the size of stage, etc.
10. When choosing your dancers, take into consideration their personality, ability, style, technique, presentation and commitment.
11. Consider lighting, props and costumes.
12. Understanding stage management is important. You need to know which is stage right, and stage left, which is upstage and stage centre.
13. Consider how your dancers will go on and off stage.
14. Avoid making negative comments such as, "Oh well, if we make a mistake no one will mind; they won't notice." That

attitude is not acceptable, nor is a badly rehearsed or presented show. Audiences can be supportive, appreciative or very critical.

15. Reflect and evaluate.
16. Accept constructive criticism; you can learn a lot from positive feedback.
17. Cancelling a performance is not an option. If you're faced with some sort of crisis, try and find another dancer or dance group that will stand in for you.

Dance Routines

Dance 'til the stars come down from the rafters
Dance, dance, dance 'til you drop.
(W.H. Auden, A. MacNeice)

Routines for groups take much practice; the timing should be spot on and the choreography creative. Choreographed routines should only be used as a guideline for those of you who want to be a solo dancer. When you can do all the transmissions smoothly you should be able to choose your own piece of music and dance spontaneously and improvise to it without having to think about your next move. Getting up and just being able to dance to any music, even if you haven't heard it before, is how dance should be.

Choose your own pieces of music for the following routines – slow, medium or quick tempos – and adapt the movements to the music.

Simple Routines

Routine 1: Slow to medium tempo
a) Do eight or 16 hip twists, or you can add the shimmy to the hip twists if you prefer as you enter onto the stage facing

your audience.

b) Spin to the right on the spot to a count of eight. Simultaneously place your right foot forward with heel raised and raise your left arm above your head, curve it gently, place your right arm down by your side and curve the arm to frame your hip.

c) Do a circle of the hip anti-clockwise.

d) Raise the left arm above your head and place hands back to back or crossed at the wrists and do a tummy roll.

e) Slowly bring both arms down and place the back of your hands lightly on the cheeks of your bottom; your arms should be softly rounded. Now do a rib cage circle or a rib cage roll.

f) Followed by two figure eights with oriental arms.

g) Place right hand gently near temple and left arm out to the side and do one grapevine to the right, followed by a camel rock.

h) Change position of arms and do one grapevine to the left, followed by a camel rock.

i) Raise arms out to the side and do two forward hip rolls from right to left, followed by one large hip circle.

j) Then repeat the two forward hip rolls from left to right, followed by one large hip circle left to right.

k) Keep the left arm out to the side and swing your right arm across you, so it's just under your bust, and do...

l) Four side steps to the right as you push your hip out to the left.

m) Sway your arms over to the right, holding them in the same position, and do four side steps to the left as you push your hip out to the right.

n) Raise your arms above your head, place hands back to back, and do eight camel rocks up on the balls of the feet, turning on the spot to the right, then eight turning to the left.

o) Bring arms down and hold them out to the side below shoulder level and spin to finish.

These routines are just a guide, as you may have to adapt the number of dance steps to go with the rhythm you have chosen. For example, you may have to do four figure eights instead of two, or four camel rocks instead of eight.

Routine 2: Medium to quick tempo
Choose your own arm movements to do with the following routines.
a) Eight travelling hip thrusts forward.
b) Four forward-step back-steps on the right foot.
c) Four hip pushes to the right, then four hip pushes to the left.
d) Eight pivoting hip pushes turning to the left.
e) Stepping back onto the flat of the right foot, do four double hip bounces travelling backwards.
f) Two camel rocks to the right.
g) Two camel rocks to the left.
h) Four camel rocks turning to the right in quarter turns.
i) Four camel rocks turning to the left in quarter turns. These camel rocks can be done either up on the balls of your feet, or on the flat of your feet.
j) Shimmy your shoulders forward to a count of four as you sway forward, then back to a count of four; repeat the shoulder shimmy sequence.
k) One step and turn step to the right with hip bounce.
l) One step and turn step to the left with hip bounce.
m) Spin to the count of eight.

Routine 3
a) Standing on the spot, shimmy your hips to a count of eight.

b) Shimmy your shoulders to a count of eight.

c) Shimmy the hips as you push to the right, then push to the left.

d) Shimmy the hips as you do a double push to the right and a double push to the left.

e) Four travelling hip steps forward (stepping to the right, then crossing with the right) – the Ghawazee step (page 160). Repeat and do...

f) Four travelling hip steps backwards.

g) Turn slightly to the left and lift and drop your right shoulder forward.

h) Lift and drop your left hip forward.

i) Slightly pivot to the right and shimmy your shoulders.

j) Follow with eight pivoting hip bounces to the right until facing the front.

k) Eight double hip bounces travelling backwards.

l) Slightly turn to the left, place right foot forward with heel raised and do four hip bounces back and four hip bounces forward with your right hip.

m) Slightly turn to your right, place your left leg forward with heel raised and repeat the sequence.

n) Turn to face the front and do four hip push shimmies travelling forward.

o) Followed by hip shimmies on the spot to a count of eight.

p) Place your right leg forward with heel raised, flick your hip up and pose.

How to Play the Zills

Everyone loves some type of music and I believe music in itself is healing. It's an explosive expression of humanity. It's something we are all touched by.

When you have mastered the dance steps and have grasped an understanding of the basic rhythms of the music, it is time to introduce the zills. The zills are small cymbals rhythmically played by the dancer or a musician as an accompaniment to the music. They are approximately 5cm in diameter with a dished centre and flat rim, and are made of brass or stainless steel.

Each zill is secured by elastic and worn just below the nail on the middle finger and thumb of each hand. When played they are struck together on the outer rim to create a light *ching* sound, and struck face to face to create a much duller sound with much less of a ring to it.

Note: Learning how to play the zills can also help to improve the flexibility of your hands and fingers.

1. When playing the zills, don't neglect your arm movements.
2. Learning to play the zills takes quite a lot of concentration so sit when practising.
3. Don't attempt to do any dance movements when you first start to practise the zills as it's a bit like rubbing your tummy and patting your head at the same time.
4. Familiarise yourself with the zills and a few basic rhythms and then combine them with a few basic steps.

Now practise the following basic rhythms. It will help if you say to yourself for example: Rt Lt ~ Rt Lt ~ Rt Rt Lt as you practise.

1) Singles 4/4 Time

Right-Left Right-Left Right-Left Right-Left

Repeat several times.

2) Basic

Right-Left-Right ~ Right-Left-Right ~ Right-Left-Right
Right-Left-Right ~ Right-Left-Right ~ Right-Left-Right

Repeat several times.

Syncopated

Right-Left ~ Right-Right ~ Right-Left ~ Right-Right
Right-Left ~ Right-Right ~ Right-Left ~ Right-Right

Right Left Right ~ Left Right Right ~ Left Right Left
Right Right Left ~ Right Right Left ~ Right Left Right

Maqsoum 4/4 Time

Variations

The two beats (right right) follow each other very quickly.
Right Right ~ Left Right ~ Right Right ~ Left Right (continue)

Right Left Right Left ~ Right Left Right Left
Left Right Right Left ~ Left Right Right Left

Saudi Rhythm

Right Right Left ~ Right Right Left ~ Right Left
Right Left Right ~ Left Right Left ~ Right Left

Kashlimar 9/8 Rhythm

Right Right Left Right ~ Right Left Right ~ Rightt Left Right Right
Right

Right Left Right Left ~ Right Left Right Left ~ Right Left Right Left ~ Right Right Right

The Veil

Dance is the loftiest, the most moving, the most beautiful of arts, because it is no mere translation or abstraction from life; it is life itself.

(Havelock Ellis, *The Dance of Life*)

There are many ways you can use the veil, which adds an entirely new dimension to the belly dance. Once you have mastered the art, your routine will be transformed into a graceful combination of undulating dance movements, enhanced by the swirling of the veil.

In the next few pages I will show you various ways of using the veil, and how to combine it with some of the belly dance movements. With imagination you will eventually develop your own creative touch and expressive moods, lending the dance an element of artistic movement, colour and mystique. However, it takes considerable practice to co-ordinate the dance steps and veil, but do persevere.

Note: Using the veil is an excellent exercise for the arms as it helps to tone up the muscles in the upper arms and improve co-ordination.

For the veil you will require a piece of light, soft, translucent fabric such as chiffon or rayon in a colour of your own choice, approximately 2.5 metres by 1 metre. If you are very tall you may need a little extra, and if short a little less.

When using the veil make sure it is not trailing on the floor. If you stand on a piece of the fabric while dancing, you may slip.

Veil Technique

How to hold the veil
Hold the veil out in front of you on the selvedge (the very edge

of the fabric) between your index finger and thumb of both hands at waist level; extend your arms along the length of the veil, then relax arms.

The floating veil

Hold the veil as instructed.

a) Twirl the veil behind you, and raise it until it is behind your head.

b) Extend your arms out to the side, then gracefully step around the room on the flat of your feet, then up on the balls of your feet. As you glide around the room, the veil should be floating out behind you.

c) As you continue to step around the room, lower the veil until it is at waist level, with arms still extended out to the side.

d) Continue to step/glide around the room and slowly and smoothly move your arms to and fro alternatively, i.e. take your right arm back as you bring your left one forward, and as you bring your right arm forward, take your left arm back.

Repeat the sequence from (a) to (d).

The butterfly

This makes an effective entrance as you turn and spin.

a) Drape the veil around your neck and make sure it's even on both sides.

b) Pinch both corners of the veil and raise your arms up to shoulder level.

c) You can also raise your arms up above your head.

The envelope

Use a light, transparent fabric; if you have chosen a fabric you cannot see through, you won't be able to see where you are going. This does happen with some learners!

a) Swing the veil behind you and drape it evenly over your shoulders so that it hangs down over your shoulders.
b) Both arms should now be on the inside of the veil.
c) Using your left hand, take hold of the two upper corners of the veil and move it over to the left.
d) Raise both arms until the veil is above your head. You should now be enveloped in the veil.
   Now do some steps and turns around the room while holding the veil in this position.

Opening the veil out

a) To open the veil out, slide your right arm across the inside of the veil over to the left-hand side.
b) Keeping hold of one corner of the veil with your left hand, take hold of the other corner with your right hand.
c) Then, extend both your arms out to the side.
   The veil should now be draped behind you, ready for your next veil movement.

The flip

a) Hold the veil in front of you on the selvedge.
b) Extend your arms out in front of you and relax elbows.
c) Flick the wrists in an upwards motion. The veil should now be resting over your lower arms.
d) Flick the wrists in a downwards motion. The veil should be hanging down in front of you.

Dance steps: with the flip

a) Hold the veil out in front of you and do four to eight travelling hip thrusts forward.
b) Flip the veil up and over your wrists and do another eight travelling hip thrusts.

The lotus

a) Hold the veil so that it is across you with the finger and thumb on the selvedge, then twirl it around so that it hangs behind your shoulders.

b) Bring your right arm across you and place it on your left shoulder.

To change position, take your right arm out to the side and bring your left one across and place it on your right shoulder.

Dance steps: with the lotus

When your left arm is extended out to the left, and your right hand is on your left shoulder, do several hip pushes travelling to the right, then change the position of your arms, extend your right arm out to the right, place your left hand on your right shoulder and repeat the dance movements, stepping to the left.

Or:

a) Hold the veil on the selvedge with your finger and thumb of each hand in front of you just below bust level.

b) Left arm should be held out to the left just below shoulder level with elbow relaxed.

c) Swing your right arm across you.

d) Hold the veil in this position as you do your hip pushes travelling to the right, then swing your right arm out to the right and hold, just below shoulder level with elbow relaxed.

e) Swing your left arm across you and hold, and do the hip push steps to the left.

The twirl

This veil movement is a little difficult at first, but a very effective movement when combined with hip rotations. When you first try this movement the veil may keep wrapping itself around your head. The secret is to keep your arms at length when twirling the veil. So keep the arms fairly straight but relaxed at the elbow when holding them up above your head and right out to the side when twirling the veil.

a) Hold the veil on the selvedge in front of you between your first fingers and thumbs.

b) Swing your right arm right across the front of you over to the left, then raise the arm until it's above your head.

c) As you bring your right arm down to the right side, raise your left arm up until it's at the side of your head.

d) Then, as you swing your right arm down across the front of you over to the left, bring your left arm down across the front of you and over to the right.

The matador

a) Hold the veil on the selvedge with the first finger and thumb of both hands across your front, just below bust level.

b) Extend your arms along the length of the veil, relax arms.

c) Keeping your right arm straight but not locked at the elbow, swing the veil across you over to the left, and raise your arm until it is behind your head.

d) Hold your left arm out to the side straight but not locked at the elbow.

To change arms:

a) Swing your left arm over to the right and raise the arm until it is up behind your head.

b) Hold your right arm out to the side, flexed at the elbow.
Now practise the following combination of dance steps with the matador veil.
When you have practised this veil movement, combine it with walks, turns and spins.

Dance steps: with the cascade

Keep your arms right up above your head with your elbows

rounded; if you drop your arms or bend them at the elbows it will look awful. The veil should cascade down behind your head.

a) Raise the veil up behind your head and place hands back to back.

b) Do four travelling hip thrusts forward with the veil in this position.

c) As you do another four travelling hip thrusts, slowly open out the veil.

d) Place your right leg forward with the heel raised.

e) As you do eight pivoting hip pushes, twists or drops turning to the left, slowly raise both your arms and place hands back to back.

f) Change feet and as you do eight pivoting hip thrusts to the right, slowly open out the veil.

g) Change feet and do eight pivoting hip pushes, twists or drops to the left as you twirl the veil above your head.

h) Then do four travelling hip thrusts forward, then four backwards as you twirl the veil above your head.

Dance step: camel rock with veil

a) Hold the veil on the selvedge with index fingers and thumbs of both hands, extend arms along the length of the veil, relax arms.

b) Hold the veil so that it is draped closely to your body.

c) Extend your right arm above your head.

d) Gather a small amount of fabric in your left hand and place the left hand on your left hip.

Note: Make sure the veil does not trail on the floor; if you step on it, you may slip and fall.

To gain the full effect of the camel rock with veil, keep the veil draped closely across your body, and your right arm extended above your head – don't let the arm drop.

a) Leading with your right foot, do eight camel rocks to the right.

b) As you change feet to travel to the left, smoothly bring your right arm down to your right hip, and raise your left arm above your head; the veil should now be draped closely across your body again.

c) Leading with your left foot, do eight camel rocks to the left. Repeat this sequence several times.

Dance step: camel rock sequence with the veil

a) Hold the veil across the front of you.

b) Raise your right arm above your head, place your left hand on your hip, and do two or four camel rocks to the right.

c) As you bring your right arm down onto your right hip, raise your left arm above your head, and do two or four camel rocks to the left.

Repeat several times until your transitions are smooth.

Dance step: camel rocks turning on the spot

Using the veil as instructed...

a) Do eight camel rocks to the right, then eight to the left.

b) As you begin your camel rocks turning on the spot, in one smooth movement, twirl the veil until it drapes down behind your shoulders.

c) After you have done four camel rocks with the veil in this position, raise both arms up above your head, place hands held back to back, and do another four camel rocks turning in the same direction.

d) As you continue with the next four camel rocks, slowly open out the veil until it is draped behind your head.

e) Twirl the veil around to the front and repeat the whole sequence in the opposite direction.

The sway

Practise the veil movement first without the step.

a) Hold the veil in front of you just below bust level on the selvedge with the index finger and thumb of each hand.

b) Extend your arms along the length of the veil, relax arms.

c) Bend your right arm from the elbow just below bust level and hold in that position.

d) Swing your left arm across you, then raise it up above your head, rounding the arm at the elbow; then push your arm back slightly so that the veil drapes down behind you.

e) Slowly take your right arm out and extend to the side.

f) Sway your right arm gently to and fro.

To change arms

Follow the instructions for (a) above.

b) Bend your left arm at the elbow and hold it just under the bust.

c) Swing your right arm across you and raise it above your head, rounding it at the elbow; then push your arm back slightly so that the veil drapes down behind you.

d) Slowly take your left arm out and extend to the side.

e) Sway your left arm gently to and fro.

Dance step: the Kashlimar with veil

a) Hold the veil as instructed above.

b) Holding the veil with your right arm under your bust, do four forward-step back-steps on the right foot.

c) As you continue to do a further four forward-step back-steps, very slowly take your right arm out to the side to below shoulder level, then gently sway the veil to and fro. Change arms and repeat the combination of forward-step back-steps on the left foot, with the veil.

Oriental drape with the head slide

a) Hold the veil closely across the front of you just below bust level, on the selvedge between your index fingers and thumbs.

b) Holding the veil fairly taut, roll your arms back from the shoulders; your arms and hands should now be on the inside of the veil.

c) Raise your arms up from the sides, until above your head.

d) Place your hands back to back and round your arms.

e) The veil should now be draped around your head and shoulders – not in front of your face.

f) While holding the veil in this position, do several head slides and head circles if you can.

When changing position from the oriental drape to any other position, with the veil, bring your arms down gracefully to the side, and smoothly – don't just drop them.

Veil 1: The shroud

Dance step: figure eights

Assume starting position for the figure eight.

a) Hold the veil on the selvedge, and extend your arms along the length of the veil.

b) Drape the veil closely across your body just below waist level.

c) Hold it in that position as you do several figure eights.

Veil 2

Dance step: with undulating figure eights

a) Drape the veil across the front of you as instructed for the basic figure eights.

b) As you do four undulating figure eights (i.e. bending your knees), slowly lower the veil until it's draped around your feet.

c) As you do four figure eights coming up, slowly raise the veil to waist level.

Practise this part of the veil sequence until you can do it

correctly and smoothly.

Veil 3

Practice

a) Hold the veil on the selvedge between your index finger and thumb of both hands, extend your arms along the length of veil, then relax them.
b) Drape the veil closely to your body at waist level.
c) Slowly raise your arms until at shoulder level.
d) Tuck your arms behind the veil (roll your arms back), then raise your arms. If you have done it correctly, the veil should shroud your head and shoulders, but not your face.
e) Slowly open out your arms and bring them down to the side until the veil is back at waist level.
Practise this veil movement until you can do it correctly and smoothly.

Dance steps: figure eights while raising heels
Practise rising up onto the balls of the feet with the veil.

a) While raising your heels, slowly raise your arms until at shoulder level, tuck your arms behind the veil, then raise your arms as in above instructions.
b) While lowering your heels, slowly open out your arms, and lower the veil to waist level.
Repeat several times until you have stopped wobbling when up on the balls of your feet.
When you have perfected your balance, try the following sequence.

Veil 4

Dance step: figure eight sequence with veil
a) Four basic figure eights holding the veil at waist level.

b) Four undulating figure eights as you lower the veil to the floor.

c) Four figure eights coming up, as you raise the veil to waist level.

d) Four figure eights as you raise your heels and bring the veil up to frame your head and shoulders.

e) Four figure eights as you lower your heels, open out your arms, and bring the veil down to waist level.

f) Practise the sequence until smooth and co-ordinated.

The mystique

a) Hold the veil on the selvedge between your index fingers and thumbs.

b) Drape it across your front no higher than shoulder level, and extend your arms out to the side.

c) Swing your right or left arm very quickly across you. The arm should now be bent at the elbow.

d) If you have done this part correctly, the veil should have flipped over your left arm and covered it.

e) Place your arm across the bridge of your nose so that only your lustrous, flirty eyes are visible.

Dance steps: walks, turns, spins

The mystique makes a good entrance, but don't forget to look at your audience and mesmerize them with your eyes as you glide, turn and spin around the room.

To remove, flip the veil from over your arm, extend your arm out to the side and position the veil for your next movement. This will take some practice to perfect so don't get too frustrated and give up.

Dance steps: with the swirl

This use of the veil looks very effective when spinning and turning.

a) Drape the veil across your front, holding the selvedge between your index fingers and thumbs.
b) Extend your arms along the length of the veil, relax arms.
c) Gather a little fabric from the top end of the veil in your left hand, and hold on your left hip.
d) Swing your right arm across and over to the left, and raise it until above your head.
e) As you spin smoothly on the spot to the right, to either a count of eight or sixteen, bring your right arm down and across you over to the right, then raise it up until behind your head.

Position of veil when spinning to the left
a) Gather a little fabric from the top end of the veil in your right hand and place on your right hip.
b) Swing your left arm across and over to the right and raise it until above your head.
c) Spin to the left to either a count of eight or six.

Ways to Wear the Veil
There are many ways of wearing the veil. Some belly dancers wear a semi-circular veil edged with sequins and semi-precious stones, secured around the neck with a clasp, which the dancer unfastens as she begins her veil routine. How you wear the veil is a personal choice, but here are some ideas which may help to inspire you. With practice you will be able to experiment and adapt your own ideas.

Some performers use Isis Wings which can look very dramatic.

Veil 1: The oriental shroud

The right side
a) Drape the veil around your shoulders and over your arms,

making sure the length is equal on both sides.

b) On the underside of the right side, approximately 15cm in from the far right-hand corner of the veil, using the index finger and thumb of your left hand, pinch a small amount of fabric, bring it up and tuck it down securely inside your waistband on the left side.

c) Your right arm should be under the veil.

d) On the upper side of the veil, approximately 15cm in from the far left-hand corner, using the index finger and thumb of your right hand, pinch a small amount of fabric, bring it up and tuck it down securely inside your waistband.

e) The veil should be under your left arm.

Having made your entrance onto the floor, you will eventually have to remove your veil without breaking the spell, which is not as easy as it looks. Make sure the veil is not twisted when you put it on or you will have problems when you remove it and not be able to proceed correctly with your next transition.

To remove the veil

a) Bring both arms in under the veil, and using your index finger and thumb of both hands, gently but firmly grip both inner selvedges of the fabric and gently pull.

b) The veil should now be out behind you, ready to use freely.

Veil 2: The sari

a) Drape the veil across your shoulders so that it hangs down in front of you. Make sure the length is equal on both sides.

b) Using the thumb and index finger of your left hand, take hold of the right inner corner of the fabric. Bring it up and it tuck it securely down your waistband on the right side.

c) Using your thumb and index finger of the right hand, take hold of the left inner corner of the fabric. Bring it up and tuck it securely down your waistband on the right side.

When you wish to remove the veil, slide both arms under the veil, take hold of both inner selvedges and gently but firmly pull.

Veil 3: The swathe

a) Evenly drape the veil over your left shoulder.
b) Take the inner selvedge of the veil on the left and tuck it down your waistband on the left-hand side.
c) Take the inner selvedge of the veil on the right in your right hand, then take the veil behind you and tuck it down your waistband on the left-hand side.
d) Both arms should be under the veil.
To remove you must use both hands at the same time:
a) Slide your left hand under the veil, and...
b) Slide your right hand underneath the veil behind you.
c) Take the selvedge between the index fingers and thumbs of your hands and pull, extending both arms out to the side.

Veil 4: Full drape

a) Hold the veil out in front of you at shoulder level, and make sure it drapes evenly.
b) Tuck it under your costume straps on the right and left shoulder so that the veil drapes down the front of you.
c) To remove: Using the index finger and thumb of both hands gently grip the selvedge, just before the tucks, and pull.

Veil 5: The wrap

a) Drape the veil around your neck, making sure the length is equal on both sides, then let the left-hand side hang loose behind you.
b) On the underside of the right side, approximately 15cm in from the far right-hand corner of the veil, using the index

finger and thumb of your left hand, pinch a small amount of fabric.

c) Bring it up and tuck it securely down your waistband on the left-hand side.

d) Take hold of the selvedge on the piece draped behind you, and tuck it into your waistband on the left-hand side.

To remove the veil

a) Take hold of the selvedge on the front piece, between the index finger and thumb of your right hand, and at the same time...

b) Take hold of the selvedge on the back piece between the index finger and thumb of your left hand.

c) Gently but firmly pull. The veil should be draped behind you.

Basic Veil Routine

As you enter the performance area, hold the veil so that it floats out behind your head.

The butterfly

a) On entrance, complete a circle around the floor as you do eight walks and four turns, followed by another eight walks and four turns. If you prefer, do four walks and two turns, followed by another four walks and two turns. (If it's a large floor area, you may have to do extra walks and turns to complete the circle.) When you have completed the walks and turns around the floor, you should be facing your audience, positioned correctly to start your next dance movement.

b) Still holding the veil behind you, spin on the spot to the right to a count of eight or sixteen. Or do eight spins to the right, then eight spins to the left.

c) Twirl the veil around until in front of you and position it for the camel rocks. Hold the veil on your right hip and extend your left arm.

d) Do two camel rocks to the right.

e) Change the position of the veil as you begin to do two camel rocks to the left.

f) Twirl the veil until it is draped up behind your head with hands back to back.

g) Do four to eight camel rocks turning on the spot. These can be done up on the balls of the feet, or on the flat of the foot.

h) As you do your last camel rock to face the audience, twirl the veil until it is draped in front of you.

i) As you begin your four hip pushes travelling to the right, smoothly move your veil over to the left. Your left arm should be out to the side just below shoulder level, and your right arm across you just below bust level.

j) Smoothly take your right arm out to the side, bend your left arm, and do four travelling hip pushes to the left.

k) As you begin your four travelling hip thrusts forward, twirl the veil up behind you, raise your arms above your head and hold your hands back to back.

l) Slowly open your arms out as you do four travelling hip thrusts backwards.

m) While still holding the veil out behind you, do eight pivoting hip pushes or drops turning to the left.

n) Continue to hold the veil in that position as you do eight pivoting hip pushes or drops turning to the right.

o) With the veil still extended out behind you, slowly lower it to waist level as you do eight shimmy hip twist walks forward.

p) As you shimmy on the spot to a count of eight or sixteen, bring your veil up above your head and place hands back to back.

q) Do two hip circles as you twirl the veil, finishing with the veil draped down in front of you.

r) Follow with four figure eights with the veil draped across in front of you.

s) Keeping the veil close to your body, slowly lower it to the floor as you do four undulating figure eights.

t) Do four figure eights lowering your heels, while extending your arms out to the side, then immediately twirl the veil until it is up behind your head with arms extended out to the side.

u) Do four figure eights while raising your heels, and simultaneously raise your arms slowly until above your head, so that the veil frames your body and face.

v) Bring your arms down to shoulder level and hold the veil in this position as you do one side step with turn to the right, then one side step with turn to the left.

w) Spin on the spot to a count of eight or sixteen.

x) As you come to the end of your veil routine, drop the veil gracefully to the floor, making sure you have placed it where you will not trip over it or slip on it during the next stage of your routine. Depending on your audience and style of performance, you may choose to flirtatiously drape the veil around the neck of a friendly spectator.

Now try choreographing your own routine with the veil.

The Stick Dance

The Egyptian stick dance has become increasingly popular with Western dancers, although there are some learners and dancers who do not like this particular dance. While undulating and shimmying, the dancer skilfully balances the stick upon her head or across her shoulders and twirls it above and below her head. It will take much practice and patience before you can skilfully combine the dance movements in harmony with the stick. The female stick dance is perceived by some as being a theatrical mimicry of the male stick dance, or the *tahtib* as it is generally known by, a competitive combative dance between two male opponents which requires great agility and skill. Supported by *mizmar* bands, they are often invited to show off their skills at Egyptian festivals such as weddings and harvest festivals.

For the stick dance, you will need a standard wooden walking stick. A piece of garden cane 1 metre in length is OK to practise with. You will also need to wear a headscarf, preferably one made from cotton or a non-shiny fabric.

Before commencing with your practice, hold the cane up above your head and swing out in all directions to make sure there is nothing you can hit, such as ceiling lights, windows, mirrors, ornaments or furniture. Quite often when learners practise twirling the cane, they lose their grip and canes go flying in all directions. Hold the stick firmly as near to the straight end as possible. It should not be held or used like a baton. The action comes from the wrists.

To familiarise yourself with the wrist action, hold your arms out in front of you and rotate your wrists to the right, then to the left, several times. Apart from when holding the cane in both hands, always hold it at the straight end, not the crook end.

Point of Balance

To find the correct point of balance before placing the cane on your head, hold your right or left arm out in front of you with your palm facing upward. Place the cane across your fingers and move it either to your right or left until it is perfectly balanced. If it rocks, it is not balanced. Before placing it on your head, assume the starting position because, if you do not stand correctly, you will find it virtually impossible to balance the stick on your head. Carefully note the central position of the stick. Pick it up at that point and place it on your head.

a) Walk around the floor until you can balance it on your head without it falling off.

b) While balancing the stick on your head, practise the hip twist walk with shimmy, and the Arabic walk; then try some travelling hip thrusts and pivoting hip thrusts.

The Twirl

Apart from when you are holding the stick in both hands, hold it at the straight end, not the crook end.

a) Raise your right arm until above your head, hold the stick horizontally and, using the wrist action, twirl the stick around as quickly as you can. Don't let your arm drop or you will whack your head with it.

b) Once you have mastered the movement, combine it with the hip shimmy.

The quicker you can do this, the more effective it looks.

The Loop

Hold the stick down by your side. Using the wrist action, push the stick out behind you, raise it up until above your head, bring it forward, drop it down to your side, then swing it back, up, then down again. Repeat several times, then try it on the left side.

Once you have mastered the loop, combine it with the following movements.

Dance step: side step with hip push

a) As you step to the right, hold the stick in your right hand and twirl.

b) As you step to the left, hold the stick in your left hand and twirl.

c) Combine the shimmy with the side step as you twirl the stick.

d) Now twirl the stick as you shimmy travelling forward, then backwards.

Horizontal Stick

a) Hold the stick at the bottom end in your right hand, and the upper part in your left hand.

b) Raise the stick above your head.

c) Bring the stick down, and hold it out in front of you just below bust level.

d) Raise the stick above your head, then bring it down behind your head.

Now combine the following steps as you use the stick.

Dance steps

a) Eight travelling hip thrusts forward, eight travelling backwards.

b) Eight pivoting hip bounces, pushes or twists to the left, then to the right.

Horizontal stick: variation 1

a) Place the stick across the upper part of your arms, raise your arms slightly.

b) Arch back and do some pivoting hip thrusts, twists or drops to the right, travelling hip thrusts, hip shimmies on the spot and travelling forward.

Horizontal stick: variation 2

a) Hold the stick in your right hand.
b) Place the stick on your left shoulder.
   This looks good with travelling hip pushes. When you change feet, place the stick on your right shoulder and hold the end in your left hand.

Vertical Stick

a) Place the hook end of the stick on the floor.
b) Place your right hand on top of the cane; make sure the stick is not leaning at an angle.
c) Rise up onto the balls of your feet, and keeping fairly close to your stick do the hip twist walk, with or without the shimmy, the Arabic walk, or the hip flick around the stick.

The Floor Dance

If you do not wish to perform the floor dance, just use the movements as a form of exercise for stretching and strengthening the pelvic floor, toning up thigh and abdominal muscles, and improving your flexibility. To protect your knees, use knee pads or a yoga mat while practising.

Note: Do not attempt any of the floor movements if you have hip, knee, neck or back problems, or had recent abdominal surgery. If you're pregnant, seek advice from your antenatal tutor.

The Descent

a) Assume starting position.

b) Stand with feet close together but not touching.

c) Keeping your weight even, extend your left leg out behind you.

d) As you bend your right knee, slide your left leg out behind you until the right knee touches the floor.

e) Bring your left leg back beside your right. You should now be in a kneeling position.

Practise this movement until it is smooth and your balance is perfect.

Arms

For hip rotations, pelvic thrusts, rib cage movements, shimmies, abdominal rolls and flutters, hold your arms slightly out to the side, elbows at waist level, palms of the hands facing upwards or downwards.

Hip Rotations

a) Kneel on the floor with your knees slightly parted, buttocks raised off the floor.

255

b) Hold your arms out to the side, the palms of the hands facing upwards or downwards.

c) Elevate your rib cage.

d) Keeping the back straight, do several hip rotations going from right to left, then from left to right.

Undulating circles

When you lower your buttocks, please keep your back straight – do not lean forward.

a) From the kneeling position, with buttocks raised from the floor and rib cage elevated, do four hip rotations as you lower your buttocks down to your heels.

b) Then do four hip rotations as you raise your buttocks.

When you first start to do these undulating floor movements from a kneeling position, you will certainly feel your thigh muscles beginning to protest. There will definitely be an "ouch" in your vocabulary! If they do begin to ache or feel a little painful, it would be advisable to stop and rest, or you may run the risk of straining your thigh muscles, and end up going up and down stairs on your bottom for the next few days!

Hip circle variation

a) Start from the kneeling position with buttocks raised from the floor and rib cage elevated.

b) Lower your buttocks down to your feet, but don't sit on your feet.

c) Push your hips over to the right and complete a large hip rotation.

d) Then, raise your buttocks and do two smaller hip rotations.

e) Lower your buttocks and repeat the sequence.

Pelvic Tilts

a) From the kneeling position, with buttocks raised up from

the floor and rib cage elevated, do several pelvic tilts.

b) To vary the movement, do four pelvic tilts as you lower your buttocks to your heels, and four pelvic tilts as you raise your buttocks. (I bet you'll be saying much more than "ouch" when doing this one!) Remember to keep your back straight as you lower and raise your buttocks.

c) Repeat four times.

Thighs aching? Then stretch out your legs in front of you and do some gentle leg stretches (see page 91).

Pelvic tilt variation

a) Start from the kneeling position with buttocks raised.

b) Elevate rib cage.

c) Lower your buttocks so they are just above your heels, hold in that position, and do several pelvic tilts. (Another big OUCH?)

Rib Cage Slide

a) Start from the kneeling position, elevate your rib cage and lower your buttocks till resting lightly on your heels.

b) If you don't get this position comfortable you may experience a little cramp in your feet.

c) Do several rib cage slides.

d) Now practise doing rib cage lifts, pushes and circles.

Rib cage slides, lifts and circles

a) Start from the kneeling position, buttocks raised, rib cage elevated.

b) Keeping your back straight, do four rib cage slides as you lower your buttocks. Practise...

c) Four rib cage slides as you raise your buttocks.

d) Four rib cage lifts or pushes as you lower your buttocks.

e) Four rib cage lifts or pushes as you raise your buttocks.

f) Four rib cage circles as you lower your buttocks.

g) Four rib cage circles as you raise your buttocks.

h) Four rib cage rolls as you lower your buttocks.

i) Four rib cage rolls as you raise your buttocks.

Shimmies

a) Knees slightly apart, rib cage elevated.

b) Shimmy your hips.

c) Now shimmy your hips as you lower your buttocks down to your heels, and keep that back straight.

d) Shimmy your hips as you raise and lower your buttocks. Repeat three or four times.

e) Buttocks raised, shimmy your shoulders.

f) Lower your buttocks as you shimmy your shoulders.

g) Raise your buttocks as you shimmy your shoulders. Repeat three or four times.
Now practise shimmying your hips and shoulders at the same time as you lower and raise your buttocks.

Abdominal Rolls and Flutters

a) Start from the kneeling position, buttocks raised, rib cage elevated.

b) Do several abdominal rolls.

c) Four abdominal rolls as you slowly lower your buttocks down to your heels.

d) Four abdominal rolls as you slowly raise your buttocks.

Back Bends

Unless you are lithe, supple, and used to more strenuous exercise, you may find back bends difficult. Back bends take a great deal of practice and mustn't be rushed as you could injure yourself. So follow the instructions carefully in the next pages. You may find it helpful to use one or two cushions, as these will give your back some support to begin with.

Back bend preparations

Stage 1

a) Start in a kneeling position, buttocks raised off the floor and back straight.

b) Take hold of your ankles and arch back as far as you can comfortably. Do not drop the head back or lift the head; hold your head in line with your back.

c) Hold for a few seconds, then come up slowly.
   Practise this several times until you feel confident and sufficiently stretched to attempt stage 2.

Stage 2

a) Start in the same kneeling position.

b) Take hold of your ankles and slowly arch back as you slide your hands up your calves; this should enable you to arch further back. Only bend back as far as you can comfortably.

c) Slide your hands back to your ankles and come up slowly. Repeat two or three times.
   With practice you will become much more flexible and be able to attempt stage 3.

Stage 3

a) Still in the same kneeling position, arch backwards and place your hands on your calves, then slide your hands up your calves.

b) As you continue to arch back, place the palms of your hands firmly on the floor by your sides and push/slide both your arms out to the sides while lowering yourself until your head and shoulders rest on the floor.

c) As you gently breathe in and out, and totally relax, your spine will sink into the floor and your buttocks will spread.

Shoulder shimmy back bend

a) Start in a kneeling position, buttocks raised, knees slightly apart and arms out to the side.

b) As you shimmy your shoulders, arch back until your head and shoulders touch the floor.

c) Come up as you shimmy your shoulders.

Back bend with hip shimmy

a) Adopt the same position as you did for the shoulder shimmy.

b) As you arch back, shimmy your hips.

c) As you come up, shimmy your hips.

Now try the back bend while shimmying your hips and shoulders at the same time:

a) While in the back bend, place your arms above your head on the floor, hands back to back or crossed at the wrists.

b) Shimmy your torso.

Back bend with tummy flutters and abdominal rolls

a) Start from the kneeling position, buttocks raised from the floor, arch back until your head and shoulders touch the floor.

b) Extend your arms behind your head with palms back to back, or with your arms raised up.

c) While in this position do several abdominal rolls, then relax.

d) Do several abdominal flutters, then relax.

e) Pull yourself up to kneeling position.

If you are flexible and co-ordinated, start your abdominal rolls or flutters as you arch back from the kneeling position. Continue the movements as your head and shoulders rest on the floor, and when raising yourself up.

Basic Upper Torso Circle

a) Kneel on the floor and lower your buttocks. Stretch forward until your head almost touches the floor.

b) Continue the body circle by swinging your upper torso over to the right.

c) Come up from the right, arch back as far as you can, then...

d) Bend over to the left, swing forward until your head almost touches the floor. You should have completed a full upper torso circle

e) To continue, swing over to the right again.
Repeat two or three times, then try it in the opposite direction, then relax.

Upper Body Circle

a) Slide your right leg out behind you, so that you are kneeling on your left knee.

b) Lower your buttocks.

c) Bend your upper body over to the left, and leading with your left arm and shoulder, stretch forward until your head almost touches the floor.

d) Continue by swinging your upper torso and left arm over to the right.

e) Bring your left arm up as you come up from the right, arch back and bring your left arm down to the side and bend over to the left to complete a circular movement with the upper torso.
Do two or three more upper body circles, relax, then try the movement in the opposite direction.

Variation

If you are feeling fit and energetic, do one large upper body circle, followed by two smaller circles.

Floor Glide with Shimmy

a) Start from a kneeling position, buttocks raised, and knees together.
b) Rib cage elevated.
c) Slide your left leg out behind you so that you are kneeling on your right knee.
d) Lower your buttocks.
e) Keep your back straight and hold your arms out to the side.
f) As you shimmy your shoulders, slowly stretch forward until your rib cage is over your right knee.
g) Continue to shimmy as you pull yourself up.

Repeat the movement two or three times, then change your position, kneel on your left knee and straighten your right leg out behind you and repeat the movement. If you are flexible enough, shimmy forward, then rise up and arch your back as much as your back will allow while shimmying.

The Snake Roll

a) Sit in the position you held for the body roll, left leg out straight behind you so that you are kneeling on your right knee.
b) Lower your buttocks.
c) Raise your right arm above your head and left arm out to the side.
d) Bend forward from your hips, bringing your right arm down until your rib cage is over your right knee.
e) Place your right hand on the floor in front of you, and gently slide your arm forward, stretching forward until your head touches the floor.
f) Roll over onto your right shoulder, bringing your left arm up so that both arms are extended on the floor behind your head.
g) Keeping your knees together, roll over onto your left side

and lower knees to the floor.

h) Using your left hand, push yourself up from the floor, bringing your right arm up above your head.

You should now be in a position to repeat the movement to the left. Try doing two or three continuous snake rolls.

The Moroccan Tea Tray Dance

The balancing act

Use an unbreakable tray. Whatever you do, don't use one that is liable to break, because when you first start to practise it will often fall to the floor. If you haven't a suitable tray, then practise with a book on your head until you acquire a suitable tray. Place your tray or book on your head and walk around the room.

Practice session 1

a) Hold your hand with the palm facing upwards towards the ceiling.

b) Place the tray on your hand.

c) Raise your arm until it is just above your head, then lower it again. Practise this a few times until you can keep the tray balanced on your hand.

d) Now take your arm out to the right side, raise your arm to just above your head, then lower it to shoulder level.

Practice session 2

Now do a circular movement with the arm:

a) Stretch your arm forward.

b) Take the arm out a little to the right.

c) Raise the arm until it is just above your head.

d) Move the arm over to the left.

e) Bring the arm down to bust level or just above.

f) Then move it over to the right.

Practise this using the left arm.

When you have perfected your balance, place four broad-based candles 7–10cm in height around the rim of the tray. If you are using a book, just use one or two candles; but please for safety reasons, do not light the candles. Then repeat the process.

This act needs a very strong neck to perfect balance, co-ordination, concentration and flexibility; and confidence to perfect and be able to perform this amazing Moroccan dance. If you are tempted to try this, tie a cotton scarf securely around your head as this will help to stop the tray from slipping.

When you have perfected your balance you should be able to walk and shimmy at the same time without the tray or book sliding off your head.

As your balance improves, add to your tray four or five broad-based plastic containers holding water. When your balance has improved sufficiently to prevent the water tippling out all over the tray, place a teapot in the centre of the tray (not a pot one as it may persistently wobble and fall off until you have perfected your balance).

Just keep practising your basic walks and shimmy walks to help improve your balance. Then gradually introduce more dance movements.

If and when you are confident enough to perform this act in public, do seek advice about using candles, as the majority of venues do not now allow naked flames for safety reasons. And don't use glue, or anything else to secure the items onto the tray; this makes a mockery of such a beautiful dance. Moroccan dancers do it with amazing skill, no tricks, and are fascinating to watch.

The body shimmy balancing the tray

a) Lie flat on your stomach, cross your ankles and practise shimmying the whole of your body for about 20–30 seconds.

b) Place the tray or book on your head and practise

shimmying until you can keep the tray or book on your head while lying on your stomach for a full 30 seconds without it falling off.

c) Now incorporate the shimmy with the snake roll while balancing the tray on your head. It is a very effective movement to do while balancing a tray of lighted candles on your head, but for safety reasons please do not attempt this until you have gained perfect balance and are in a safe environment supported by safety experts.

The lift

Practise this first until you are able to do it smoothly, then do it balancing the tray on your head.

a) From the kneeling position, lower your buttocks and gently sway to the left and down onto your left buttock.

b) Place the palm of your left hand on the floor beside your left knee, your right hand gently resting on your right knee.

c) Place the weight on your left hand, and raise your right arm up to just below the tray.

d) Simultaneously raise your left buttock, straighten your right leg.

e) Hold for a few seconds.

f) As you bring your right arm down, simultaneously pull your body up from the left, relax your right leg and come up to a kneeling position.

The ascent

When you have finished your floor dance you must ascend gracefully, and smoothly.

a) Come up onto both knees into the kneeling position.

b) Place your right leg slightly forward, so that the right foot is flat on the floor and your knee bent.

c) Slowly and gracefully raise yourself, and place your left leg beside your right leg. You should now be positioned to go into your next dance step.

Arms

Now practise your ascent with the arms:

As you raise yourself up from the floor, bring your arms up from the sides and place them on either side of your head, with your elbows bent and hands pointing towards the ceiling.

If you decide to include the floor dance in your repertoire, with or without the tray, choose movements you can do with ease and feel comfortable with. Some dancers only perform the back bend from the kneeling position and include a few shimmies or abdominal rolls before ascending.

Conclusion: This Sacred Dance

When a woman dances this sacred dance, this beautiful art, through its natural rhythm and stream of life, she expresses and celebrates her divine femininity, embraces the awakening of her feminine consciousness, her creative energy, her sexuality, her fertility.

When a woman dances this sacred dance, this beautiful art, she has the potential to find empowerment, celebrate the veneration and communication of the divine feminine, and restore harmony, happiness and contentment.

When a women dances this sacred dance, this beautiful art, she unites humanity with the great mother earth, the sacred feminine, and symbol of life, death and rebirth. She restores balance and harmony with the universe, renewing life's forces, nurtures and nourishes.

When a woman dances this sacred dance, this beautiful art, she is a woman reborn, full of passion and love, who understands life and her inner feelings. She will embark on a new journey, a joyous passage of enlightenment, inspire passion, and unity, to love all things, and be at one with the world.

(Tina Hobin, 2012)

AYNI
BOOKS

"Ayni" is a Quechua word meaning "reciprocity" – sharing, giving and receiving – whatever you give out comes back to you. To be in Ayni is to be in balance, harmony and right relationship with oneself and nature, of which we are all an intrinsic part. Complementary and Alternative approaches to health and well-being essentially follow a holistic model, within which one is given support and encouragement to move towards a state of balance, true health and wholeness, ultimately leading to the awareness of one's unique place in the Universal jigsaw of life – Ayni, in fact.